Up the Down Hill

Up the Down Hill

One woman's struggle to survive major depression

Rozanne W. Paxman

Writers Club Press
San Jose New York Lincoln Shanghai

Up the Down Hill
One woman's struggle to survive major depression

All Rights Reserved © 2001 by Rozanne Warner Paxman

No part of this book may be reproduced or transmitted in any form or by any means, graphic, electronic, or mechanical, including photocopying, recording, taping, or by any information storage retrieval system, without the permission in writing from the publisher.

Writers Club Press
an imprint of iUniverse.com, Inc.

For information address:
iUniverse.com, Inc.
5220 S 16th, Ste. 200
Lincoln, NE 68512
www.iuniverse.com

ISBN: 0-595-16787-X

Printed in the United States of America

Foreword

While reading "Up the Down Hill," I started having memories of a book that impressed me in high school: "The Odyssey" by Homer. From almost the first page of Rozanne's book, I had the feeling that she, like Homer, was taking me on a journey—an odyssey of healing that was personal, at times intimate, and even sacred. As she faced and dealt with each new problem or obstacle and shared her understanding of herself, I had the sense that she was simply reporting, in a candid and clear way, the truth—the truth about her journey. I respect her honesty in this book.

Depression and despair have been compared to the bubonic plague of our time. The victims of this plague are numerous, much more numerous that warranted by our knowledge of how to treat it. In the last few decades, there has been considerable progress concerning the different kinds of depression and what can be done to prevent and ameliorate their disturbing and destructive effects. Many books have been written by professionals that are truly helpful. As a mental health professional, I—for one—have wished that a broader audience could somehow be reached with the hopeful news that depression is treatable and that it is no longer necessary to be doomed to a life wishing one were dead. "Up the Down Hill" may well reach an appreciable portion of those and help them begin the climb up and out.

Recent research has demonstrated that religious individuals are not more depressed than the population at large, as many have supposed, but they do have stress and burdens peculiar to the kind of responsibilities they shoulder, as well as emotional and spiritual resources to deal with those responsibilities. One of the important benefits that came to Rozanne during her "breakdown" and plunge into depression was her heartfelt need to make the most of her spiritual resources as a believer of Jesus Christ. She rediscovered the power of her faith to keep her alive, to solve her problems, to keep her trying, to inspire her, to develop her gifts and talents, and to do the many things required to continue her journey.

There are often misunderstandings about depression in a religious community. There are those who claim that all mental health problems can be resolved with enough faith and that disorders like depression are a sign of spiritual weakness. Fortunately, these kinds of misguided views are diminishing. An increasing number are recognizing that depression can be rooted in any combination of causes, including inherited biochemical disorders, dysfunctional ways of thinking, stress and pressure, abuse and trauma, lack of purpose and meaning in life, and yes—sin and unbelief. "Up the Down Hill" frankly describes one woman's struggle to face and deal with the unfolding realities of her life, in order to overcome her depression and obtain happiness.

This book is a gift to us all. Most of us, in some way, have been touched by the hand of depression, whether within ourselves or through the association of those we love. If you suffer from depression, "Up the Down Hill" may help you in your journey. It may help you find strength, begin needed changes, start restoring a relationship, or commit to not giving up. You may discover within yourself the light, put there by God, which is a reminder that He is there and He will see you through the challenges of this life journey.

Larry Beall, Ph.D.
Director, Trauma Awareness & Treatment Center

Preface

This story is true. I have, out of concern for the privacy of the many people that are mentioned in this book, changed some names and details. Additionally, I have tried to change enough life and story details of the people I met in the hospital to secure their anonymity. I didn't feel that it was proper for me to infringe on their privacy. The picture I paint of life in the hospital is absolutely correct and I would say that the majority of things you will read during this section of the book are true. The secret of which details have been changed and which details have not been changed will remain with my fellow in-patients and me until the end of time.

To my fellow in-patients, I would like to say that I hope this book meets with your approval. The five days I spent in the hospital with you were absolutely critical to my recovery and all of you taught me valuable lessons. I learned to love each of you and have often wished that I had kept in contact with you. I hope you are all doing well. You will forever remain in my heart. May God bless you with health, love, and happiness.

So here we go. I'm opening and baring my soul to the whole world. Please, take my gift and use it kindly.

Introduction

Even Good People Get Depressed

I am pretty ordinary, really.

Just like most people, I have strengths and weaknesses. I've made my share of mistakes, but I've also had my share of successes. While I've done many stupid things, I've also made a lot of good decisions as well. I've never had extraordinarily terrible things happen to me.

I was fortunate enough to be raised in a good middle-class home by two parents who loved and cared deeply for me. I was taught the Gospel of Jesus Christ through the efforts of my parents and auxiliary teachers and gained a strong testimony during my fourteenth year. I had siblings who both loved and squabbled with me, just like many, many other women. I had a good education. I married a returned missionary in the temple and after many years of struggling, was blessed with four beautiful children.

So then, just how did I find myself struggling with a deep, dark depression that was so devastating to me that I often found myself suffering through the days in a supreme effort just to stay alive? How did I get there and, more importantly, how did I recover? These are the questions I will attempt to answer. For while I was involved in the contest of my life, I searched in vain for something to read that was written by someone like myself.

I wanted desperately to read a book written by an ordinary, faithful, active Latter-day Saint woman because, while I could find an almost endless source of excellent books by experts, I wanted to know what someone like myself had gone through and how they managed to survive it. I wanted reassurance that even though I was tormented in this terrible way, I could recover—that there was hope for me at the end of this long journey I unwittingly found myself on. I wanted to know that other active Latter-day Saint women had experienced major depressions and that it was possible to fully recover and maybe, even become stronger because of the experience. I wanted hope. I longed for it. I thirsted for it like a wilting flower longs for a cool drink of water.

Our Latter-day Saint society is still rather closed when in comes to this topic. Members feel afraid to say they are suffering depression. They are afraid they will be seen as weak minded or sinful. They dread hearing someone tell them to either "Pull up their bootstraps and get on with it" or that "if they just had a strong enough testimony of Christ they wouldn't be depressed!" Major depression just isn't a "good" Sunday lesson topic. I knew that there had to be members around me that had either gone through it or were currently experiencing the same thing, but I couldn't seem to find them. I felt so cut off from everyone. I thought, "If there was only a book written by someone like me." So in the end, after the stormy clouds had finally passed, I decided to try and write the book myself.

Please don't misunderstand. I don't consider myself an expert on depression. There are many, many things I don't understand about it. But I do know this; I know how it feels for me, Rozanne Warner Paxman, to be in the dark regions of major depression. I know how it feels to be convinced, even temporarily, that everyone you love would be much better off without you. I know how it feels to pray to be able to withstand it just this one more moment. And I know how it feels to be at the very darkest hour of your life and have someone throw out the all-important life raft that pulls you back into reality. I now know that even good people—with strong testimonies of the restored gospel and of Jesus Christ—can suffer depression, major depression.

So please forgive me if my experience differs from yours. Please forgive me if my recovery doesn't follow the same path as yours has or will. These differences don't mean that your experience is not valid or your path to wellness is not as sound. Just as we all suffer in our own way from this disease, we all find our unique way out of it in the end. This is simply my story, put into words with the desire that I may help someone by sharing my experience.

The important thing for us all to know is that there is hope. There are wonderful doctors and treatments available to us now. There is assurance in the gospel and there is healing available to us all from the great Physician, Jesus Christ. Life can be sweet again and peace can be restored. Joy can be felt and days can be met with anticipation instead of dread. We can become whole once more.

So I dedicate this book to you, my fellow travelers to the land of despair. I dedicate this book to you with the prayer that it somehow is able to relieve even the smallest portion of the pain you are feeling or have felt. I dedicate this book to you in the hopes that your loved ones, friends, neighbors, and brothers and sisters in the gospel will gain empathy for the struggle you are facing. I dedicate this book to you with all my love.

Rozanne W. Paxman

The Hospital

Day 1

▼

The door banged. "Wake up, now. You can't sleep all day."

Rozanne blinked as the curtains were pulled open and the light from outside came streaming in the window to the right of her bed. To add insult to injury, someone turned on the overhead light and abruptly, she felt thrust into an unknown world.

"Where am I?" she thought to herself. After a few moments it registered, "Oh, I remember now…the hospital."

Her eyes traveled around the room in an effort to acquaint herself with her surroundings. The room was medium sized, set up much like a college dorm room. There were two single beds built into the wall with bookcase headboards. Each had a nightstand to the right and a closet over a bank of drawers built into the wall on the left. The only desk in the room, which was under the sole window, had already been claimed by the other occupant of the room. This person, for the moment, was unidentified, as there was a blanket pulled over her head.

"I need to go to the bathroom," she mumbled.

"The bathroom is through that door," the reply came back.

This interchange brought her attention to the individual that had stunned her into awareness. As if her mind had been read she heard, "I'm Mark. I'm on the floor today. Do you need anything else?"

Without saying anything, she stared back at him. He must have been about 21 years old, but he looked younger. He was tall, had wavy, light brown hair, blue eyes, and those good looks normally associated with someone who is the "All-American-boy-next-door" type.

Mark continued, "I know this is all new to you. You'll find some personal supplies in the bathroom. When you are through, come on down the hall and we'll show you the ropes. You're on red for now. That means that we need to know where you are at all times. Don't worry though, I'll help you to learn what you're expected to do. See you in a minute."

Mark looked over at the other bed in the room, "Laura. Laura! Time to get up. Breakfast is in half an hour. Group starts at nine. You need to go today."

There was no movement from the occupant of the other bed, but Mark didn't seem to take notice of this. Smiling at Rozanne, he turned and walked quickly out of the room. After he left, she grabbed her shoes from under her bed, shoved them on her feet, and stumbled into the bathroom.

She groaned when she caught sight of herself in the mirror. Her short blond hair was standing straight up. She had mascara rubbed under her eyes which, she was dismayed to see, were bloodshot and spotted with purple specks all around the outside because of the broken blood vessels caused by the river of tears she had cried the night before. Her skin was pale and blotchy. Her mouth felt dry and fuzzy.

"Ugh," she moaned. "Just great, Rozanne, just great. Never thought you'd end up here, did you?"

She spotted a harvest-gold plastic container that held shampoo, conditioner, soap, toothbrush and toothpaste and a comb. She hurriedly went through an abbreviated, sloppy version of a morning routine. At this point, her appearance was the last thing on her mind. She was concentrating on shutting out the emotions that were begging to be felt. She didn't want to cry. She didn't want to lose it again. She had to maintain. She *had* to maintain. She had to…

Rapidly, she strode through the two doors that stood in her way to the hall. She needed to get out of the bathroom. She didn't want to be alone…not today…

Down the hall to the right, she spotted the nurses station. It was a large cluster of rooms with two entrances and a long desk built beneath a bank of sliding glass windows that separated the staff from the patients. She could see Mark inside, talking to a girl with long, brunette hair and a man with curly hair and a salt-and-pepper beard. The man was dressed casually, much like someone attending a baseball game, and wore silver wire-rim glasses. He seemed to be listening closely to the longhaired girl, who looked very much like a hippie-throw back from the 1970's because of the clothing she wore and the leather hair-clasp holding her hair back from her face. The girl seemed to be very excited about something. Her hands were flying about the room as fast as her mouth was moving.

Mark spotted Rozanne and motioned for her to join him. The other two asked him a question and then turned to a large white-board on the wall behind them. When Rozanne got closer to the window, she could see that the board had a column of patient names with information—such as doctors' names, medications used, and dietary needs—written to the right of the them. She quickly found her name and noticed that she was identified as red in the status section, and her doctors were Manning and Beall. No one else had two doctors.

"I wonder why…Does this mean I'm worse than anyone else here?" she mused.

Mark smiled at her as she reached the end of the hall. He slid open the glass window and asked, "You ready?"

She nodded and as he slipped out of the door, he directed her attention towards a poster on the wall.

"This is the patient status hierarchy chart. You can see that there are three levels: red, yellow, and green. You're on red now because you're new. All patients are on red when they first get here for at least twenty-four hours. How are you feeling now? Do you feel safe?"

Rozanne knew that he must mean, "Do you feel like killing yourself today?" Since that seemed to be too much effort at the moment she replied, "Fine."

"Good. If you keep feeling that way, I'll talk to your doctor about moving you up to yellow. Then you'll get to go down to the cafeteria for meals. You'll like that better. When you're on red we have to keep you in line of sight continuously. If you need to go to the bathroom, you'll need to tell one of us first. You'll eat your meals in the day room. Basically, you'll need to stay close to staff at all times. Later, when you're on yellow, you can go to your room when you want and have freedom of mobility. Green usually happens right before you go home. When you're on green, you can take charge in community group meetings and go outside on the grounds by yourself. Do you have any questions?"

She shook her head, so he continued, "Let's go on a little tour, okay?"

Mark led her into a medium sized room that had two large, leather couches with end tables covered by magazines, a large, blue, circular table surrounded by chairs, a small refrigerator, a television set and VCR in a cabinet and again, a large white board on the wall. This time the whiteboard was empty. Rozanne noticed that there was a glass window on the wall between the nurses' station and this room.

"To watch us," she thought. "I feel a little like Shamoo at Sea World."

"This is the day room." Mark stated, "This is where you'll take your meals while you are on red. They ought to be bringing up your breakfast any minute. If you smoke, the area that patients use is right out that door. You'll have to ask before you use it. Do you smoke?"

"No."

"Okay. Let's go into the other room. It's the room on the other side of the nurses station."

They walked the twenty-five feet to their destination and she noticed that the only remaining possibility was to enter the hall where her room was. There were approximately ten rooms positioned on both sides of this hall. At the end of the hall stood a large set of locked double doors.

"I guess I won't be running away," she thought.

Mark continued his oration. "This is the room where patients attend group counseling sessions. You'll be here with all of the other patients from our wing. First, you'll have community group. Community starts at 9:00. That's when you discuss any group issues that may be on people's minds. You'll set your goals for the day during this group as well. At 10:30 we have therapy group with Rhaun. He's the guy with the beard you saw in the nurses' office. Then at 12:00 you'll have lunch and at 1:30 you go to substance abuse group. You look surprised. I know you aren't here for that, but all patients have to go to it. It's okay, though. You'll find that they talk about things that can help you, too. Recreational Skills are taught from 4:00 to 5:00 with dinner following. Visiting hours are from 7:00 to 9:00 every evening. Then at 9:30 we have community group again and after that you can go to bed, if you want. Don't worry about remembering everything because there are plenty of people around here to make sure you know what to do next. It's important that you go to all of the groups. You won't be able to move up the levels if you don't. You have to make an effort to get better. You'll be fine, though. I'm sure you'll do well. What do you do for a living?"

"I'm a junior high teacher."

"Really! My sister teaches junior high, too."

"Where does she teach?"

"North River Middle School."

"Oh, no!" Rozanne groaned. "I used to teach there. I just transferred at the beginning of this school year. Who's your sister?"

"Deb Johnson."

"Deb's your sister?" Rozanne said, smiling as she remembered. "Oh, that's great. She's such a neat girl! Everyone just loves her. She's so bubbly and fun."

Her eyes flew wide open as the realization hit. "Oh, no…You've got to promise me that you'll never tell her you saw me here. I'd just die if anyone found out that I'm here. It's so embarrassing!"

Mark reached over and placed his hand on her shoulder. "Don't worry about that, Rozanne. You'd be surprised at how many people I meet here—prominent people in both the church and the community. Your problem is more common than you realize. No one likes to talk about it so people generally don't find out someone is here—unless the patient wants them to know, of course. No one can call you unless they have your code number. If anyone calls here, we won't even confirm that you're here unless you've specified that you want him or her to know. We try very hard to maintain confidentiality because it's so important to our patients. It's too bad that it has to be that way, but we understand how our patients feel."

Rozanne relaxed. She was surprised to learn that Mark was Deb's brother. They didn't look at all alike. Deb was extremely tiny with very dark hair and eyes. She studied him closely and as she did, she began to see the family resemblance. He and his sister shared the same gleam in their eyes. No wonder she had immediately liked him.

"I'll leave you now," Mark continued, "Breakfast is here and you'll want to eat it before it gets cold. Don't feel shy about asking us for help, if you need it. See you later."

Mark turned and went back into the nurses' station and Rozanne went back over to the day room. When she arrived, she saw that the two people in the room were already eating and were in the middle of a discussion about coffee creamers.

"I have a right to like anything I want to," announced the thin woman. "Besides, lots of people like milk in their coffee. It's not peculiar at all. Sweetened condensed milk—now that's peculiar!"

"Yuck!"

Suddenly the two women noticed that they were not alone in the room, "Who are you?" the heavy woman said. She had frizzy, dirty, light-brown hair and a round face with two double chins. The clothes she was wearing were as disheveled as her hair. The woman picked at the hospital-issued footsies on her feet and stared at Rozanne suspiciously. "Are you new staff?"

The thin woman answered for me. "Oh, don't be ridiculous! Anyone can see that she's a patient. Don't let Macie bug you. She doesn't mean anything by it. I'm Heather," she continued, smiling. "I've been here for six weeks and I'm still on red. Sometimes I feel like killing myself, but I won't lie about it like the others do. I've got to get better this time, so I'm not playing games. That's why when I feel like hurting myself, I go right up to staff and tell them. Some people won't admit it. They're the ones that people ought to worry about. They're just kidding themselves, though. You can't pretend this away. Are you here for depression or abuse?"

Rozanne contemplated Heather's question. She'd never had anyone talk to her like this before. "Depression," she answered.

"Oh. Us, too," nodded Heather. "Macie has been here before, haven't you, Macie? She was here for two weeks, went home for one day, and then checked herself right back in. Got home and couldn't handle it. Pretended that she was better. Didn't you Macie—pretend that you were better?"

Macie shrugged her shoulders and tore a milk carton open. "Yeah.... Yeah, I did that. Only I didn't know that I was pretending then. I just figured out what they wanted me to say and do and I did it...Went home...Only problem was my husband was there. He wanted to know why I hadn't done his shirts the last two weeks...His shirts...Then he leaves. I'm in the psyche ward for two weeks and he never comes to see me, even once! I come home and he asks me about his shirts and then leaves to go off with his buddies and so I thought to myself, 'Macie, you ought to go back there before you really hurt yourself this time'—so I did.

Came right back and checked myself in. Quit lying to myself. My life stinks and now I know it. Only problem is, now I don't know how to get myself out of this mess without killing myself to do it. You know...my mother told me that she regretted having me. "You're a mistake," she said. "A mistake. I wish you'd never been born," she said...."

"Save it for group." Heather interrupted. "Macie does that...She'll go on and on and on. Say, what's your name? You didn't tell us."

"Rozanne."

Heather patted the chair next to her. "Well, Rozanne. Sit down. Do you want to eat? Breakfast is here, although it's not very good. It never is. Today we're having sausage, eggs and toast. There are all kinds of juices and milk, and stuff like that, in the refrigerator. Help yourself to whatever you want. Don't like the food much myself, but the juice is good."

Rozanne took the chair next to Heather and opened the lid of the breakfast tray. It looked...interesting.

"Do you want your sausages?" Macie said, "I just love sausages. I'll eat your sausages, if you don't want them. I just love it when we get sausages for breakfast. We don't get them much. I'll eat yours, if you don't want them."

"Macie, shut up," demanded Heather. "Leave her alone. Let her eat her own sausage if she wants to. Rozanne, you'll have to watch that. She's not supposed to eat other people's food, but she still tries to get it away from you when she can."

Rozanne began eating her breakfast mindlessly, studying Heather as she ate. Heather was really quite pretty. She was about 5'5" with long, black hair and big, dark, sad eyes with lots of eyelashes. Her hair was arranged in a big clip on the top of her head and the white sweat suit she was wearing complimented her complexion. There was a kind of easy grace about her that Rozanne thought surprising. She certainly never imagined meeting someone like Heather in a place like this.... She never imagined that *she* would be in place like this.

When they were through eating, Macie and Heather got up from the table. Heather disappeared down the hall somewhere and Macie plopped herself on the couch and began thumbing through an ancient issue of Cosmopolitan.

The hippie-throw-back girl entered the room carrying a large, red binder. She took a chair from the table and pulled it directly in front of the couch, sat down, and flipped through the pages in the book. "Macie, it's time we set your goals for the day." she instructed. "Tell me, how are you feeling right now?"

Macie held the magazine up in front of her face and answered from behind the pages, obvious indifference ringing in her voice. "I feel sad, confused, anxious, and bored."

"Is that it?" asked the girl, as she wrote down Macie's reply in the binder.

Macie turned a page in the magazine. "Yep."

"What are your goals for the day?" the girl asked.

"My goals?"

The girl sighed impatiently and tapped her pencil on the binder. "Your goals."

After turning another page in the magazine before answering, Macie finally complied, "I guess I want to work in my anger packet today and I'll read some of the information Rhaun gave me yesterday after group." She lowered the magazine slightly so she could glare at the girl. "Is that enough?"

"I'm concerned that you don't seem to be challenging yourself," the girl answered. "Do you think that you can come up with any goals that could address your bigger issues?"

"My issues?"

"Yes." The pencil began tapping again. "The circumstances that brought you here." The tapping stopped. "Macie, you know all of this. Why do we have to go through this every morning?"

"My husband is my issue," Macie said angrily. "You know, when I went home all he wanted to know about was his shirts...His shirts! Never a "How are you doing?" or nothin'. His shirts..."

"Macie, try to stay focused here," the girl said. "I want you to think about coming up with issues that *you* can control. You can't control your husband's reactions. You can only control yourself. Try to come up with some goals that will help you make the changes *you* need so that *you* can be in control of your own life. Do you think you could do that?"

"No."

"Macie. You've got to try."

"It's too hard, Mattie. If I just had a different mother...Why doesn't my husband come to see me? We've only been married for two months. I just don't understand it."

Mattie leaned forward and patted the round leg closest to her. "I certainly can appreciate the pain you must be feeling, Macie. Maybe you could use that pain to focus on some goals that can help you overcome the feelings of helplessness I hear you expressing. Could you try?"

"Oh, all right." Macie said, barricading herself behind the magazine pages again. "I'll think about it."

Mattie sat back in her chair triumphantly. "So, I'll write down that one of your goals is to think about developing specific ideas that can help you move toward becoming more in control of your own life. Is that all right?"

There was another pause as Macie turned a page before she surrendered with a grunt.

"Thanks, Macie. Have a good day and good luck with your goals."

Mattie moved the chair closer to Rozanne. "Hi. I'm Mattie Walker. I'm one of the counselors on the unit. How are you feeling today?"

"Okay, I guess."

Mattie found a blank form in the book. She wrote Rozanne's name at the top of the sheet and then looked up again. "What emotions are you experiencing?"

"What do you mean?"

Mattie smiled brightly at her before replying. "One of the things we ask people to do here is to put labels on the emotions you are experiencing. I know it might seem strange to you at first, but do you think you could try?"

Rozanne began chewing on a hangnail nervously. "Well, I guess I could try."

She tried to *feel*. It was hard. She had spent most of the last two months trying to shut off her feelings and her body didn't want to let it happen. She felt terrified that if she started to feel again, she would lose control—like she did last night. Feelings were scary—especially bad feelings.

She had been carefully taught all of her life that she was supposed to feel happy, grateful, and loving. These were appropriate emotions. Sadness, discouragement, frustration, anger, and emotions like these were not appropriate. They were emotions to be turned off—like a spigot on a water jug. Just turn them off and don't let them out. Keep them in that jug and don't let them escape. Good girls don't feel unhappy or discouraged. They are grateful and happy that their lives are as wonderful as they are. Just think how much better your life is than some other unfortunate soul. It could be worse. Oh, those emotions just make you feel guilty. Bad...

She felt a tap on her hand. "Rozanne, are you all right?" Mattie asked.

"What..." Rozanne said, jumping slightly. "What?" She looked up to see a concerned look on Mattie's face.

Mattie searched Rozanne's face with her eyes. "I was afraid I lost you there for a minute."

Rozanne looked away. "No. I guess I was just thinking."

"That's obvious." Mattie said. "What were you thinking about? You began to look upset."

Rozanne shifted in her seat as she struggled to answer. "About feeling," she replied, studying her hands. "I'm not sure I can let myself do it. I may fall apart again."

"It's all right, Rozanne. We are here to help you through this."

Rozanne bit her lip and began. "Well…I guess I feel afraid."

"Good," encouraged Mattie.

Rozanne sighed and continued. "…And nervous. I don't know what to expect here. I'm afraid of this environment. I never thought that I could come to a place like this." She looked up at Mattie. "Am I safe here? Is this going to ruin my life that I needed to come here?"

Mattie wrote in her binder a moment before replying. "So—do I hear you saying that you feel concerned about your future?"

"Yes, I guess so…Can we stop now?"

"Okay," Mattie said, "Now that you've done that, we ask you to make some goals for yourself for the day. Do you think that you could do that?"

Rozanne didn't quite know how to respond to this question so she said, "How about I just have the goal to try to figure this place out and what I'm expected to do while I'm here."

"I think that's an appropriate goal for your first day," Mattie replied. "Thanks, Rozanne…Have a good day and good luck with your goals."

Mattie got up from the table and left the room. When she was gone Macie threw the magazine on the floor and blurted out, "She bugs me…She really bugs me."

Rozanne had completely forgotten that Macie was still in the room. She looked over and saw that Macie was studying her closely. "So—are you a Mormon or what?"

Rozanne felt the air rush out of her lungs. "As a matter of fact, I am. Why do you ask?"

Macie shrugged and said, "I'm a Mormon, myself. I've even been on a mission. Can you believe that? Yeah, I know I look bad right now, but I don't think I've always been that way. Maybe I was and I just didn't know it. You look like a Mormon. You look, oh, I don't know…sort of squeaky…"

"Squeaky?"

"Yeah. You know, squeaky—like squeaky clean," Macie said. "I can tell that you're a mess right now, but I'd be willing to bet that you've never done anything real bad. Yup, you look squeaky. It sort of yells out, "I'm a Mormon." I can tell, you know. I can see 'em comin' fifty feet away. There are several of us here, right now. Heather—she's a Mormon. She's not squeaky, though. She's had some hard times, but you'll hear all about that later. Gloria is a Mormon, too."

"Gloria?"

"You'll see her in group. She's on yellow now, so she's gone down to the cafeteria for breakfast. She's been on a mission, too. She's not like me, though. You'll find out. She's *different*."

Different...
"Rozanne, you know that we're different than other people in this town."

"Why, Mama. Why are we different? I don't want to be different. Miss Golding said that we need to try to get along with each other. I try, Mama, but the other kids don't want to talk to me. They tell me that I'm different because I'm smart and I play the violin. They think it's not good to be different. I want to be the same."

"Rozanne, sometimes it's good to be different. Did you know that Grandma was an actress when she was young? She even got asked to go to California with a touring group that came through town. The leading lady got sick and your Grandma was asked to fill in for her. She did so well that they wanted her to continue touring with them. She could have gone to California and been an actress."

"Yes, but Mama, she didn't go, did she? She didn't want to be different. She wanted to be the same."

"It's not a bad thing to be smart, Rozanne. It's not a bad thing to be able to play the violin."

"But the kids tease me, Mama. They tell me I'm weird. They don't like me. Nobody plays with me at lunch. It's a bad thing to be smart. I want to be the same."

"Rozanne. Rozanne! Are you listening to me?"

"Huh?"

She looked up to see Macie squinting at her. "You looked like you went somewhere."

"No, it's all right." Rozanne sighed. "I guess I was just thinking…"

Macie was offended. "Well, I guess so. Hey, I can take a hint!"

They were interrupted as Mattie quickly strode into the room. "Ladies, its time for group. Rozanne, do you know about community group?"

"Yes. Mark filled me in on it."

"Good." Mattie pointed towards the door. "Well, shall we?"

As they entered the group room, Rozanne could see that they were not alone. By the left wall there was an oblong table surrounded by chairs. Heather was at this table and was engrossed in coloring a picture.

There were two others coloring as well. One was a stocky, tall Spanish-American boy, with closely shaven black hair. He looked to be about eighteen and was wearing baggy blue jeans an enormous blue shirt and was laughing at something the other girl had just said. She looked as if she was in her mid-twenties. She had medium-brown, waist-length hair and was wearing tight jeans and shirt. They were so engrossed in their conversation that they didn't even seem to notice that someone had entered the room.

Curled up in a fetal position on the love seat to the right of the table was a woman with medium-light-brown hair who appeared to be in her thirties who was clutching a small photograph to her chest. She looked like she had been pried out of bed because she was still in her well-worn pajamas and robe.

Against the back-wall was a long couch that matched the love seat. Macie promptly took up position at the far-left corner of this couch, tucking her right leg under her torso, dangling her left leg over the edge. She sprawled her arms out along the side and back as far as they would go, in a successful effort to claim as much of the couch as was humanly possible.

At the opposite end of the couch was a middle-aged man with dark-blond hair and a mustache. He was holding his head in his hands when they entered the room, but sat up and weakly smiled at Rozanne when she looked at him.

There was a long, brown leather couch against the far right wall. A girl with dark-brown, curly, shoulder-length hair who appeared to be in her mid-twenties was totally engrossed in writing in a red, paper folder. She was sitting crossed-legged in the center of the brown leather couch.

After considering where to sit for a minute, Rozanne sat as far to the right on the leather couch as she could manage, trying to distance myself from the other occupants. She wondered if one of these women could be her roommate, Laura.

Mattie pulled a big, leather chair from the far end of the table over to the open end of the U-shaped formation that the couches formed and sat down. "How is everybody this morning?" she began.

There was no response.

"Gloria, how are you feeling this morning?"

The girl on the couch by Rozanne answered without looking up. "I feel tired and anxious and sad and confused."

Mattie wrote Gloria's responses down. "Thank you, Gloria. What are your goals for today?"

"I want to do ten pages in my anger packet and write in my journal."

"Is that all?" Mattie asked.

"That's it."

"Well, have a good day and good luck with your goals." After writing something else in her binder, Mattie turned to the man on the couch with Macie. "Hi, Andy. How are you doing this morning? Has your stomach settled down?"

Andy grimaced. "A little better. I'm still pretty shaky."

Mattie nodded at him. "That's to be expected. You only came in last night and it usually takes a good thirty-six hours for the physical symptoms to go away. Can I help you with anything?"

"No." said Andy in a soft voice. "Thanks. I guess I'll be all right."

"Andy, could you try to tell us how you are feeling this morning?"

Andy looked confused. "Didn't we just do that?"

Mattie shook her head a few times. "Not really. We just talked about your physical symptoms. I'm asking about your emotions now. I know that it may be hard for you. It's common for people with substance abuse problems to shut off the emotions they are feeling. Can you try to figure out how you feel emotionally?"

"Oh. I guess so." Andy answered. "I guess I feel anxious…I really want to make it this time. I want to quit. I hope I'll learn some things here that will help me, but I'm afraid it really won't make a difference. I also feel bad about how I've treated my family. I used my drinking as an excuse to ignore them."

"Great, Andy." Mattie encouraged. "That's a good start. Now, what goals do you have for the day?"

"I guess I want to do some thinking about my life," he said, "and to try to figure out what I can do to make things up to my family. I also need to figure out what I'll do with myself after I leave here. I don't want to fall back into the same old patterns that caused me trouble."

"Andy, I can tell you've been thinking about this. Have a good day and good luck with your goals."

"Thanks," said Andy, relief ringing in his voice.

Mattie scooted her chair until it faced the left side of the room and watched the group coloring at the table for a moment, as if she was deciding what to do next. Directing her comments to the longhaired girl with her back towards her, she asked, "Lizbeth. How are you feeling today?"

Lizbeth stopped coloring and tossed her head. "Mad and angry and about ready to rip the curtains off of the window. I'm not supposed to be here. I'm supposed to be in the day program, but my stupid insurance company made me come here. I want to get out of this dump."

Mattie began writing in her binder furiously. "Wow! You're not happy. Do you have any goals for the day?"

Lizbeth pulled a face. "I want to get hold of my doctor and get this mess straightened out."

"Is that it?" Mattie said as she wrote.

Lizbeth turned back to her project. "That's all I'm in the mood for."

"I can see that." Mattie finished writing and then studied the young man. "How about you now, Colby? How are you feeling today?"

The boy looked up and smirked, "Cool. I've only got twenty-three more days in this joint."

"Colby..."

Colby swept his arms out in the air. "Oh.... I know," he said in an affected tone. "*Feelings*. Okay. I FEEL bored. I FEEL sleepy. I FEEL bugged. I FEEL!"

Colby and Lizbeth started laughing hysterically. Mattie simply watched them and then continued, "Heather, how are you feeling today?"

Heather gave Colby and Lizbeth a dirty look that quickly had the effect of quieting them back down. They buried their heads into their coloring projects in an effort to control themselves. After she could see that they had managed to do it, she began, "I feel sad...I feel confused...I feel...anxious. I'm trying to get a handle on my grief today. I want to just let myself feel it. For so long, I have made myself stay so busy that I haven't let myself feel the pain. This scares me a lot, but I am going to try to do it. I'm going to write my thoughts in my journal and read some chapters in the book Carol gave me about grief. I guess that's it."

Mattie smiled at Heather and said softly, "Thanks, Heather. I think you've done very well. Have a good day and good luck with your goals." She wrote Heather's information in the binder and then said loudly, "Hey, Tawny...Tawny! Are you going to talk to us today?"

The curled up woman on the love seat grunted.

"How do you feel today?"

Tawny curled into a tighter ball as she muttered, "Tired."

"Tired…" Mattie said. "Okay. What are your goals for today?"

Tawny pulled the edge of her tan bathrobe over her face. "I want to go home to my son."

Mattie put down her pencil. "We know that, Tawny. What goals are you going to set that can get you closer to going home?"

Tawny pulled the bathrobe higher and the photograph closer. "I want to go home."

Mattie shook her head impatiently and insisted, "What goals, Tawny?"

Tawny flipped over on the couch and rolled back into a tight ball with her back towards Mattie. "My goal is to go home today."

Mattie let out a long, soft sigh. "Okay, Tawny. Your goal is to go home today." She closed her binder and put it under her chair. "Let's go on to something else now. Does everyone know Rozanne?"

The group at the table said at the same time, "Hi, Rozanne."

"Hi." Rozanne replied, disappointed that there didn't seem to be a Laura in this group, which made her even more curious about her missing roommate. Why wasn't Laura here?

Mattie went on, "What community issues do we have to talk about this morning?"

Macie began bouncing as she shouted, "Oh, I have one! I have one! Can I take a turn now?

Mattie replied, "Yes, Macie. You have been rather patient this morning. Okay. Tell us, what is your issue?"

Macie grinned. "Well, let me see. Oh, yeah. I remember now. It really bugs me when *some* people get candy from their visitors and then *some* people won't share with the rest of us. *Some* of us don't get visitors much. It makes us feel left out. It's not *my* fault my husband never comes to see me. You know what? He never even calls me. No one comes to see me much. I call my bishop and he just says that I'll have to schedule an appointment through his executive secretary. He's too busy for me, too. He said I should forget about the shirts. My husband only cares about his shirts. My mother said she didn't want me.…"

"Macie." warned Mattie. "Try to stick to the subject, please."

"Sorry."

Mattie leaned back in her chair and folded her arms across her chest. "Let me see if I understood you. You feel left out because you don't have many visitors and your feelings got hurt when Heather didn't offer you any of her candy that her children brought to her last night."

"That's it! *Some* people don't share."

Mattie looked towards the table. "Heather, what are your feelings on the subject."

Heather shifted in her chair and pulled her clip out of her hair. After she had rearranged her clip back into her piled up hair, she replied, "It was my understanding that Macie wasn't supposed to eat candy because of her health problems. That's the reason I didn't offer her any. I thought she knew why I couldn't give her any of it."

Mattie looked back towards the couch, "Macie, what about what Heather is saying? Does this help you understand why she couldn't offer you any candy?"

Macie sat as still as a statue as the group waited for her response. Finally Mattie asked, "Macie, do you wish to add anything else to the conversation."

"No."

Just then Mark stuck his head in the door and motioned to me. "Rozanne, your doctor is here to see you."

Mattie smiled at her. "Go on. We'll see you later."

As she entered the hall, Rozanne spotted a man she assumed was her doctor. He was in his mid-forties and was dressed much like a college professor in dark-green corduroys, a white, striped shirt, and a dark, wool, herringbone jacket with suede patches on the sleeves. He had a dark complexion with black hair. Turning when he heard the door open, he held out his hand and said, "Hi, Rozanne. I'm Larry Beall. Margaret told me a lot of nice things about you."

Dr. Beall led Rozanne down the hall a few steps and opened a door on the left side. It was a small room with three chairs and a small, rectangular table on one side. He took the chair at the far side of the room and she sat down in the chair opposite him.

"Rozanne, why don't you tell me about what brought you here last night?" he began. "Margaret has told me a little bit, but I'd like to know what you think."

"I just lost it, that's all," she answered, with as little emotion as possible. "I was in the closet crying and it scared my husband, Gary. He called Margaret and they agreed that I should come here. I was tired of fighting it by myself, so I came."

"I'd like to know more."

It had been a long two months. Her fifth period choir class was the worst group she had ever dealt with since starting to teach in 1987. She wanted them to learn to read music and to sing songs that weren't on the radio and they didn't like it.

The battle commenced on the very first day of school. There were angry challenges to every statement or idea Rozanne offered.

One day, one of the most belligerent girls of the group walked out of class— just simply stood up and walked out of the choir room—and went home. Rozanne turned in a referral to the office, as this was a serious offense. She was surprised to learn later that no punishment was assigned because, as the Vice-Principal had put it, "I talked to her and she agreed not to do it again."

Rozanne went to the councilors for help. "Please, this class is too full," she begged. "Fifty-two students—when at least half of them are problem kids—are simply too many. There aren't enough places to spread the problems around the room. How can I play the piano for them to sing and watch them at the same time? It isn't right. It isn't safe. Please, help me!"

The response was always the same, "Sorry, there's nowhere else to put them."

The stress she felt began to emerge as physical symptoms. She started to have chest pains, especially after climbing the stairs at school. She never had any symptoms at home, just at school—even though she hadn't figured this out yet. One morning, the pains got so bad that she couldn't breathe. When she called her physician to make an appointment, his nurse told her to go to the emergency room immediately.

At the emergency room, the doctor ordered an EKG, which came back with odd-looking results. As a result, the emergency room doctor decided to send her to a cardiologist for further tests. When the tests the cardiologist administered came back as normal, her doctors scratched their heads and decided to see if she had an ulcer or gallstones. Those tests also came back negative and everyone was stumped. The pain was real—they'd seen it—but what was causing it?

One day a girl in her 5th period class decided to "flip-the bird" at Rozanne, using her right hand to "roll" the middle finger of her left hand up and down, up and down. An aide, whose sole purpose in the room was to help the resource kids (students with learning disabilities) with their written work, witnessed the offensive finger movement. After the class was over, the aide reported to Rozanne that the girl did it over and over every time she looked down or turned her back to the class. Rozanne had no choice but to write out a referral on the incident for the Vice-Principal's intervention. When, after two days, she hadn't hear anything about the matter, she searched the halls for Mrs. Jepson. At last she was discovered supervising the lunch crush in the cafeteria.

"Abbey, did you see the referral I sent up on Mandy?" Rozanne asked, once she arrived at her side.

"No," Abbey replied, shaking her finger at a student across the room.

As Rozanne began filled her in on what had happened in the classroom, Abbey shifted her attention from the students to me, "That's an automatic suspension! I always give a two-day suspension to any student that makes that gesture towards a teacher. I'll call her in after lunch and talk to her and then I'll get back to you."

During the last period of the day Mandy and her friend, Janielle, came storming into the room, demanding to talk to Rozanne about the referral. When she pointed out that she was teaching a class at the moment, Mandy became loud and combative, so Rozanne asked the class to read a section in their books and escorted the two girls into her office. "Mandy, this is not a good time to talk about this," she said, once was closed behind them. "I'd be happy to discuss it with you after school."

"Mrs. Paxman, I didn't do it." Mandy whined. "You're just making it up."

"Mandy, you know that I didn't see what you did," Rozanne replied. "But there was an adult aide in the room that day and she witnessed the whole thing. What reason could she have to make it up?"

Mandy looked over at her friend and they rolled their eyes at each other. "Come on, Mrs. Paxman. I didn't mean it. It doesn't mean anything, anyway."

"I may be much older than you are," Rozanne sighed, "but I've known what that gesture meant since I was five years old. We'll talk about it later. Right now, you need to go back to your class and I need to teach the class that's waiting for me. Goodbye, Mandy."

Mandy and her crony stormed out of the room leaving Rozanne to deal with the questioning looks of her current class.

After school, Rozanne decided that she would try to slip out of the building. She wanted to avoid another confrontation with Mandy. "Let the VP deal with it..." she thought. "That's her job." Rozanne decided to leave the building from an exit she didn't normally use. The ruse didn't work; she ran smack-dab into Mandy and her mother. "My daughter would never do such a terrible thing," the offended mother said. "What makes you say that she did it? You must have it in for her."

Mandy stood by her mother's side with an expression on her face that said, "Got ya now, Mrs. Paxman."

Rozanne's heart began to pound. "How about we take this inside?" she suggested. "I'm sure that Mrs. Jepson would like to be part of this discussion. Would you please follow me?

Rozanne led Mandy and her mother down the hall and, fortunately, found Mrs. Jepson in her office. "Mrs. Jepson," Rozanne said with that "Help me, *please!"* look on her face, "Mandy and her mother would like to have a conversation about the matter I referred to you. Could you see us now?"

"Sure, come on in."

"Mrs. Jepson," Mandy's mother began after they were seated, "I certainly don't understand what all of this is about. I talked to Mandy after you called me and she has assured me that she is innocent of this charge. She feels that Mrs. Paxman doesn't like her and is trying to get her thrown out of choir."

Abbey turned to Rozanne and said, "Mrs. Paxman, I've spoken to the aide this afternoon and she assures me that what you told me is true. Could you please explain to Mandy's mother what the aide saw Mandy do in choir that day?"

Rozanne obeyed Abbey, demonstrating the gesture that Mandy was reported to have made. After watching the short demonstration, Mandy's mother exclaimed, "Well! I certainly don't know what that gesture means. Even if Mandy did do it, I'm sure that she doesn't know what that means, either. I think that you should just forget all about it."

Abbey and Rozanne exchanged meaningful looks and Rozanne said, "I think it may be helpful for you to understand what I've been going through as a teacher with this class." She then went on to explain the challenging class periods, the questioning of every assignment and song, the behavior problems, the subterfuge that had been going on during the six weeks that had passed since the beginning of the school year.

Abbey jumped in and said, "I think I should tell you something that even Mrs. Paxman doesn't know. Several of the students have admitted to me that there is a large group that is united in their efforts to drive Mrs. Paxman out of Southland. They don't like the fact that she is making them learn something. They think that they should just "hang out" in choir—that it should be a sluff-off class. This class is hard for her to deal with. I believe that peer pressure motivated Mandy to make that gesture to Mrs. Paxman."

The mother turned to her daughter and asked, "Is this true, Mandy?"

"Yes. I guess so," Mandy answered sheepishly.

"Mandy, your dad and I have always taught you that you shouldn't go along with the crowd when they are heading the wrong direction. You remember that, don't you?"

"Yes I guess so."

"Will you promise that you won't do it again, Mandy?"

"Yes. I guess so."

Abbey sat back in her chair and triumphantly smiled, "It looks like everything's settled. Mandy has promised not to do it again. Thanks for coming in."

Rozanne looked at Abbey in amazement. It had happened again. There would be no suspension. There would be no consequence. It was just, "Be a good girl and don't do it again." "What do these kids have to do before the administration will do something about it?" she wondered. "Kill someone? Start a riot?"

After Mandy and her mother left the room, Rozanne asked, "Abbey, would you do me a favor? I'd like to show you my list of students for this class. I don't think you understand what I am facing. Would you come back to my room with me?"

"Sure. I'd be happy to. "Abbey replied.

They walked silently down a long hall, descended the three flights of stars and traveled down another long hall to Rozanne's room. Rozanne got the role sheet from her clipboard and handed it to Abbey. As she read the names on the list, Abby's face started to twist as she exclaimed, "Oh no! She's a brat. Oh, that's a tough one, too. He's a regular one in my office. So is she…And her…and her…and him, and him and her…" Abby looked up at Rozanne and said softly, "I didn't know."

"I've been trying to tell you. It's hard…so hard."

"Yes. It would be. What can I do?"

Her hopes rising, Rozanne said, "Could you do me a favor? Would you talk to the counselors about not sending me any new students? It's bad enough now, but I keep getting two or three more every week. I can't keep going like this."

Abbey nodded her agreement. "I'd be happy to. You definitely have more than you can handle here. I'll talk to them myself."

That was a Friday. On Sunday night Rozanne felt suicidal. It was the third Sunday in a row that she had felt that way since the first of October.

It wasn't that she really wanted to kill herself—she loved her family and knew she had a lot to live for—it was just that she felt so trapped. She had a contract. She had to complete the school year. If she didn't, she wouldn't ever be able to teach in Utah again. School districts don't look favorably on teachers that quit in the middle of the school year. It was just so hard to go to school, day after day, and face all of that animosity with no back up from the administration. She was working incredibly hard—ten to twelve hours a day. So many students…So much to do…Such anger from her 5th period class…

She struggled with herself all day to make the decision to go back there. She had always loved teaching. How could she deal with hating it now?

Monday came too soon. The day went mercifully well until the 5th period class came in. The room buzzed with excitement and Mandy grinned like the proverbial cat that ate the canary. The word of Mandy's triumph had quickly spread through the school. Everyone in that room knew that Rozanne couldn't do anything to them, no matter what. There was no threat of consequence for poor behavior. The kids were on their way to victory.

One girl walked up to Rozanne and whispered to her, "Mrs. Paxman, I just want you to know that you are my favorite teacher. I don't care what everybody else says." She showed Rozanne her leg. She had written "Mrs. Paxman rules!" in blue ink on her thigh.

"Thanks, Julie. I appreciate it more than you could know."

As the class progressed, the student's behavior slid quickly downhill as they were trying their best to set her off to get some "evidence" to use against her. Although, at one point she was tempted to leave the room, in the end she managed to get through the longest forty-five minutes of her career.

After they left she was shaking. "I've got to get out of here," she thought, "I need some help to deal with this."

She decided to make an appointment with an Employees Assistance Program counselor. This was a program the school district participated in to make psychological counseling available to employees and their families. She went in the private phone room and dialed the phone.

"Hurry, hurry, hurry. Pick up. Pick up"

"E.A.P.," said a young sounding voice. "Can I help you?"

"Hello. This is Rozanne Paxman from Mt. Alta School District. I'm in trouble here and I need to make an appointment to talk with someone."

"Could you hold a moment?" inquired the voice.

"Yes, but hurry," answered Rozanne. "I have less than three minutes before my next class begins. I have to get back to my room."

After a while, an older sounding, female voice said, "Hello. How can I help you?"

"This is Rozanne Paxman from Mr. Alta School District. I'm having some trouble coping with my situation at this school and I need to talk with someone. Could I make an appointment?"

"Okay." answered the voice. Rozanne heard a sliding sound followed by the sound of pages flipping. "How about Thursday at 4:30?"

Rozanne's son had a doctor's appointment at that time, so she answered, "I can't come then. Is there another time?"

The voice paused and Rozanne heard a page turn in a book. "Well, how about tomorrow night at 7:00?"

Rozanne sighed. She had to play the piano for homemaking meeting during that time. "I'm sorry—I have a prior commitment. Is there another opening?"

"You aren't making this easy," the voice said in an annoyed tone. "When can *you* come?

Rozanne started to feel panicky. She should have brought her day planner with her. "I'm so stupid," she thought to herself. " I'm sorry." Rozanne told the voice. "I'm having a hard time thinking. I've got to get back to my room. I've got a class waiting for me. I've got to get back."

"You aren't being very cooperative," the voice said sternly.

"I don't mean to be that way. I've just got to get back to my class and I can't think now. Can I call back after school today?"

The voice let out an exasperated sigh. "Oh, all right. But are you all right now. Are you safe?"

"Safe?" Rozanne asked.

"Safe." replied the voice.

Rozanne wasn't quite sure what the voice meant, so she answered, "I guess so. Listen, I've got to go. I'll call later."

She managed to get through the rest of that day somehow. As soon as she got home, she called E.A.P. back. This time she couldn't get through to the original woman she had talked to. A different person talked to her and said that they couldn't get her in until that Saturday.

"Saturday! Saturday!" Rozanne cried. "I really need to see someone sooner."

"I'm sorry, but we're all booked up now," the new voice said. "Peter has some time on Saturday. You can see him then."

"That's too long," Rozanne thought to herself. "But I don't have a choice. I have to see someone…" After a moment, she relented, "Oh, all right. I'll take that time then."

When she hung up the phone, she was overcome with an escalating feeling of panic. Saturday! She couldn't wait that long. Facing those kids tomorrow was her pressing concern.

She decided that she'd call her son's therapist, Margaret. He had been seeing Margaret since the previous spring and Rozanne trusted her. She'd call Margaret.

Margaret responded to her immediately and scheduled an appointment the next morning. She told Rozanne to take the day off. "Just tell them that you need to see the doctor."

Rozanne knew they'd buy that one, because of her "mystery pains" and so she made arrangements for a substitute.

The next morning found her sitting in Margaret's office. She felt comfortable there. Margaret was about Rozanne's age, had dark hair and eyes, and they shared similar interests. She even had some of the same problems Rozanne had with her children. Her office was filled with an overstuffed country couch, cheerful prints on the walls, and knick-knacks and toys that would appeal to the children she worked with.

Margaret was like her office. She wore clothing that gave her patients a comfortable feeling—like you could rely on her. As Margaret entered her office and saw Rozanne's face, she exclaimed, "What's going on, Rozanne? I've never seen you this upset."

Margaret watched Rozanne closely as Rozanne told her what had been happening at school. She wrote a few things into a file folder and then set the folder on her desk. Rozanne could see in her expression that she was carefully considering what to say.

"You know what I want you to do?" Margaret began, "Take the rest of the week off. Tell them it's doctor's orders." Margaret nodded to herself. "It is, you know. You've got to pull yourself back together before you go back into that classroom again. I'll see you again on Thursday. You've already got that appointment with Peter at EAP on Saturday. Go to movies. Sleep in. Read a good book. Think about your choices. We'll talk on Thursday. I want to think about what I can do to help you."

Rozanne went home and followed Margaret's advice. It felt great not to have to go back to school. She could almost pretend that she never had to go there again.

On Thursday, Margaret met her with a big grin on her face. "You know what you're going to do today? You're going to play in the sand."

Rozanne laughed at that. "Play in the sand?"

Margaret nodded at her with a twinkle in her eye. "Play in the sand. You're going to make a sand tray picture. Let's go in the back room."

Margaret took her down the hall into a room that was lined with shelves. The shelves held every kind of small object imaginable. Rozanne could see dragons, animals, trees, rocks, toys, cars, figurines of people doing different things, buildings, abstract objects—and lots more. On a large table were three, large, plastic trays filled halfway with sand. One tray had white sand, one had brown sand, and one had dusty-pink sand.

Margaret told Rozanne to get a basket and fill it up with any objects that caught her eye. She instructed, "Don't think about it. Just pick up anything at all that you like—that feels right. I know it sounds crazy, but it really works. Don't worry about it. Just do it."

Rozanne walked over to the shelves and started looking at the contents. She giggled. "This feels stupid."

Margaret answered, "I know. Do it anyway."

"Okay," Rozanne agreed, "but it makes me feels dumb."

Some figurines that are used in miniature Victorian Christmas villages caught her eye. There were lots of them. There were even some people that could be used for any season of the year. She began choosing...

First a figurine of a blond-haired girl reading a book went into her basket with another figurine of a little girl washing dishes. These were followed by figurines of a mother and a little girl sitting in a chair together, a grandmother sewing a dress, and another grandmother holding the hand of a little blond girl.

Finally, she began choosing figurines that would complete the picture. She choose a lamp post with a red bird sitting on it, three large trees that looked like they could be apple trees—one with a tire swing hanging from it—a Christmas tree, and a fireplace. When she was finished, she looked over at Margaret. "Now what do I do?"

Margaret pointed at the trays. "Pick a sand tray. Look... We painted the tray bottoms blue so you could have water if you want. This is all natural sand. This pink sand comes from the Caribbean, I think. Pick one and then put the things you've chosen in the sand. Arrange them any way that feels right. You'll know what I mean when you start playing with them."

Rozanne picked the tray with the pink sand and began placing the objects in the tray. She moved them around a little and then announced, "I'm finished."

"Are you sure?" asked Margaret.

Rozanne looked around the room again and studied the scene she had made in the sand tray before answering. "Yes, I'm sure."

Margaret looked at the sand tray for a while, then pointing at the grandmother who was sewing a dress, she asked, "Tell me about her."

"I guess that's my Grandmother Stevens," *Rozanne replied after thinking for a moment.*

"You loved her, didn't you?" *Margaret said.*

"Yes, I did. She died right before Gary and I got married. She was great. I saw her almost every day of my growing-up years. She was almost like a mother to me."

"Only better, huh?" *Margaret added.* "Grandmothers have some freedom with their grandchildren that their mothers don't have."

Rozanne looked at her with surprise. "I've never thought about it before," *she said.* "I guess you're right. I just know that I felt totally loved and accepted in her house. She loved me no matter what—no strings attached. Me—warts and all."

"Sounds like you felt safe with her," *Margaret said.*

"Yes, I did. I miss her. I wish she was here and I could sit on her lap." *Tears began filling Rozanne's eyes. Margaret handed her a tissue and then asked,* "Rozanne, have you noticed something about your sand picture? All of the people you picked are women."

"I noticed that myself as I was choosing the figures," *Rozanne replied.* "It just felt right."

"I'd like you to think about why you did that," *Margaret said.*

'I don't know..." *Rozanne said, shrugging her shoulders.* "Maybe it is because I always felt happy when I was around my Mom and Grandma. I think I feel envious of them, too. While their lives weren't easy, their roles were clear. They had enough time at home with their children. They had time to garden, sew, and spend time doing things they felt were important."

Rozanne looked away from Margaret's gaze. "I feel like I'm drowning. In fact, I often dream that I am drowning. I'm in the ocean—far away from shore. I feel myself sinking down...down...down...I reach up with my right hand—trying to get it above the water. I can feel myself stretching up as high as I can go. I'm trying to get someone, anyone, to pull me out of there and prevent me from dying. Sometimes I even wake up with my arm sticking straight up in the air. The dream seems so real. It's not difficult to figure out what that means. I feel overwhelmed by my life and don't see anyway out."

Rozanne wiped her eyes and blew her nose. Margaret asked softly, "How are you feeling right now, Rozanne?"

Rozanne wiped her eyes again. "I guess I feel sad...kind of confused, too. I still have the same problems that I had on Monday, but I don't feel like I'm going to fall apart this minute. I feel like I can get through the next few days, anyway."

"Good." Margaret said. "So you'll be all right until you can see Peter at E.A.P.?"

Rozanne picked up her purse off of the floor. "Yes. I'll be all right."

The next few days flew by in a blur. Rozanne wished that she could grab them and hold onto them like you would a small child who was about to run out onto a busy street. It felt far too dangerous to move ahead.

Saturday arrived and Rozanne went to Peter's office. She asked her husband, Gary, to drive her there because, this time, she felt threatened by the counseling appointment. Peter was an unknown.

When they were entering the building, they ran into a man that identified himself as Peter. "Hi! I'll bet you're Rozanne Paxman," he said, stretching out his right hand in greeting. "Is this your husband? Great! Hey, I'm glad you're a few minutes late, too. I had a little trouble getting away from home this morning."

Peter was in his early thirties, had light-blond hair and a beard. He was dressed casually and seemed relaxed, which made Rozanne feel less nervous. After unlocking the building and his office, he ushered them in, seated Gary in the reception area, and took Rozanne into his private office to talk.

"Why don't you tell me about yourself?" he began.

Rozanne sighed. It was hard retelling the problem. "I guess I ought to tell you about why I think I'm here, right?" she said.

"That's a reasonable place to start." Peter agreed.

Rozanne told him the story of how she got to Southland Junior High, what had happened to her since starting there, and how she was feeling. When she finished he asked, "Just how married are you to being a teacher? It sounds to me like maybe you ought to look at doing something else."

She shook her head forcefully. "You've got to know something, Peter. All I've ever wanted to do—my whole life—was to be a music teacher. When I was in junior high, my band teacher and my violin teacher had a significant influence on me and I decided that I wanted to be just like them. They made me believe that I could achieve anything—if I just tried hard enough. They got me through those hard years. They were very hard."

"What do you mean?" asked Peter.

Junior High was like a nightmare for me. The other kids... They didn't like me because I was different. I was smart. I played a lot of musical instruments. My parents owned one of the only department stores in town and the other girls were jealous of my clothes. I matured early, which created problems as well. One time, some of the other girls threw me down in PE and hit me in the chest while screaming, "You'll get breast cancer! You'll get breast cancer."

Peter's eyebrows shot up. "Really?" he asked.

Rozanne nodded and continued her story. "I didn't know how to handle it and I didn't respond well. I know that finally I reached a crisis point with it all. I was tired of feeling like the scapegoat of my group—that was my purpose, you see. The girls I hung around with just tolerated me because I was fun to tease."

"A lot of kids feel that way," said Peter.

"I know," Rozanne replied, "but I made things worse than they needed to be. One day I committed the ultimate "sin." I sat with a different group of girls as lunch. Then I compounded the problem by yelling at the "ambassador" who was sent to inquire about my treasonous behavior. I got so upset that I ran home and refused to go back to school for two weeks. This worried my mother so much that she went to the school and complained to the principal. He responded by calling the girls into his office."

"Oh, no!" said Peter. "I think I see where this is going..."

Rozanne sighed and nodded at him. "Mom finally managed to get me to go back to school. When I entered my first class the kids erupted in sound. There were catcalls, hoots, and worse coming at me from every side and the teacher did nothing about it. Nothing at all... The rest of my years were, basically, just like that. A lot of the teachers didn't seem to do anything about it. Some of the teachers were very nice, but I didn't feel safe in many of those rooms."

Peter frowned at her as he asked, "Rozanne, did you say you were in junior high when most of that happened to you? Doesn't that strike you as odd that you'd be teaching junior high? Did you know what you were doing when you began teaching that age group?"

"I thought you'd pick up on that," she answered. "I guess in some ways it is odd, but I did it on purpose. I always felt like some of the teachers could have done a better job handling the situation and I wanted to see if I could make things better for kids. I love junior high kids. I've always done especially well with them, until *this* one *class*, *this* one *year*. I don't understand why I can't get things turned around in that class. I don't understand why I feel so miserable teaching school now."

"That's a question that we need to look at," he answered. "Tell me, were there any other factors in your life that could be causing you problems?"

"I was sexually abused, one time, as a child. I remembered what happened about twenty years ago, but I think I've handled the memories of the incident rather well. I don't think that it should be considered an issue now. We've had some major financial problems during our marriage," she told him. "But my husband and I are very close and have been able to handle things well, together. We do have some "interesting" kids in our home," she laughed, "but there are probably people that have much worse. No," she said with emphasis. "I think that this issue over my teaching is what is causing my major problem at the moment."

Peter looked up from his note taking. "So, your relationship with your husband is good?"

Rozanne smiled, remembering, "Actually, it's better than good. I've been blessed this way. Gary is my best friend."

"How did that happen?" Peter asked her with a puzzled tone of voice. "Usually someone that has had some of your experiences ends up marrying an abusive husband."

Rozanne shrugged her shoulders. "Just blessed, I think."

Peter shook his head in disbelief. "I can say that you've done at least one thing right in your life. You married well."

"Yes, I did."

Peter put down the folder and pen and rocked back in his chair. "Rozanne, I think I can help you. It ought to just take us three or four months. How do you feel about working with me?"

"All right, I guess. You seem nice. Yes, I think it will be all right—if I can just get through next week."

Peter pulled out his appointment book and looked through the pages until he found the right spot. "How about I see you again on Tuesday night?" he asked. "Then we can talk about what we'll do next."

She got through the rest of the weekend pretty well. Sunday night was still pretty scary, but she knew that she just couldn't keep staying home. It was like what you always hear about getting back on that horse. The longer she put it off, the more intimidating it would become. So she decided to take a big breath and "dive back in those waters."

When she entered her classroom on Monday, she gasped. She had expected a mess because that usually happened when she had a substitute, but this time it *looked even worse than she expected. Quickly, she went to work and managed to get it in order before the first bell rang.*

The morning classes went rather well. They usually did, though. Her other classes were great kids. There were a lot of them—one class had sixty 7th graders in it, but they loved her and the feeling was mutual.

Around 10:30 a messenger from the office arrived. Rozanne looked at the pink slip and learned that she was expected to go to the office immediately.

She didn't like that. She had always made it a practice never to leave her students alone. How could she keep them safe if she did? But the message had indicated an emergency, so she decided that she better comply. She gave the students a task to work on, slipped across the hall and asked the band teacher to keep an eye on her class, and ran to the office as quickly as possible.

When she entered the office, the secretary Bobbie looked up at her, "Oh, Mrs. Paxman. I didn't mean for you to come up right now."

"But the message said it was an emergency!"

"Oh yeah, right." Bobbie said, snapping the wad of gum in her mouth. "Well, you know, we got a message from the District Office. It seems that you were over paid this year by $900."

Bobbie stopped chewing and glared at her suspiciously. "Didn't you know that you were getting too much? You should have known. How come you never told us that your checks were too high?"

"They were too high?" Rozanne gasped. "The checks seemed about right to me. I knew that we were supposed to be getting a nice raise this year. This is only my second year working for this district. The raise I thought I had was about what I was used to seeing when I taught in California. I didn't see any reason to ask about it."

Bobbie tapped her foot irritably. "Well, this is not California! It seems to me that you should have known. You're just lucky that we discovered it now. If this had continued until the end of the school year, you'd have owed the district thousands and thousands of dollars. Then what would you have done?"

Rozanne felt the walls of the office closing in on her and the stares of the office personnel burning holes in the back of her shirt. "I—I—I don't understand" *she said.*

At that precise moment, principal walked out of her office. "Bobbie, what is going on?" *she demanded.* "Why is Mrs. Paxman up here now?"

Bobbie looked at the principal with an innocent expression on her face. "I called her up here—you know—about the money that she was overpaid. She's got to pay back the district. They want to know what she's going to do about it."

The principal looked at Rozanne sternly. "Rozanne, did you know you were getting too much money?"

"Of course not!"

The principal relaxed and said, "Bobbie's right about one thing. You'll have to take care of this. You should have known that your check was too high."

Rozanne was still confused. How on earth could this have happened?

The principal waved her hand impatiently. "Never mind. Look—you can go over to the district office after work to straighten all of this mess out. You better go back to class now."

As Rozanne walked back to class she shook with fear. "Too much money? How did it happen?" *she mourned.* "Why did they act like I knew about it? Why did this have to happen today?...And it's fourth period. Guess what class is coming in next? THAT class. Oh, dear. How can I get through it?"

She remembered something that Peter had told her to do. She was to imagine that junior high girl that she once was and then imagine that she was holding her in her arms and assure her that everything would be all right. Rozanne tried. She tried. But she was so shaky. So shaky...

BUZZZ!! Rozanne jumped. "Oh, no! There's the bell. They'll be coming now. They'll be coming. What will I do? What will I do?" *she thought in alarm.* "I know. I'll try to get them singing right away. Maybe I can get them singing and they'll leave me alone today. Maybe it will work. I've got to get through this day. I've just got to."

The 5th period class entered the room yelling and shouting at each other while pelting her with questions. "Where were you last week? Why weren't you here? Why did you stick us with that substitute? What an idiot! Did you know that he held us in from lunch for five minutes? I bet you told him to do it, didn't you? What an idiot! Why weren't you here? Were you faking it or something? Bet you had a heart attack, huh?"

Rozanne managed to get them quieted down and seated correctly. After checking their theory pages, she asked them to pull out their Christmas music. She knew that they tolerated Christmas songs.

They began singing. Rozanne took them through all of the sections of the song "Christmas Yule," group by group. They practiced their parts. They went over the breathing and the words. They did everything that she could think of that didn't require her to play the song's accompaniment on the piano.

She hated that she had to play the accompaniment for them. There weren't any students in this class that could play the piano well enough to help her. That meant that there had to be times during each class period when she couldn't watch them and with this class, that definitely was not a good thing!

Finally, the moment arrived when she had *to get behind the piano, but with only ten minutes left in the class, she thought she'd be safe. They began singing the song, with Rozanne at the keyboard. When they were on the third refrain, out of the corner of her eye, she saw two chairs suddenly switch places. This immediately caught her attention because students were not allowed to move the chairs around. She had her room set up so that there were three distinct sections; each with color-coded and numbered chairs. It was part of her discipline technique and was a very powerful tool. The kids knew the rules; no one moves the chairs in Mrs. Paxman's room without her permission.*

She quickly determined who had moved the chairs and asked the offender to go to the practice room for the rest of the class period. She'd talk to him later. They continued practicing the song until the bell rang. One of the sopranos immediately stormed up to her and said angrily, "Mrs. Paxman. You've got to get Jeff to quit spitting. He was spitting all over and it was so gross! It about made me hurl!"

By this time the chair-moving offender, Larry, had left the practice room and had joined them. He added, "Yeah, Mrs. Paxman. It was so gross. Look what he did." Larry pulled a chair from the second row down in front of her and pointed at the seat. It had a six-inch pool of spit in the middle of it. On the left side was a long dribble of snot. They were right—it was gross.

Rozanne was puzzled. Why on earth would Jeff do something like this? He was usually so quiet. There were a few good kids in this class, and he was one of them. "Jeff. JEFF..." she called to him. "Would you mind coming down here? I'd like to speak with you for a minute."

Jeff slunk over to her and as he got closer, she could tell that something was wrong. He was foaming at the mouth...Foaming...She'd never seen anything like it before. And there was that snot again. This time it was hanging down from one nostril. It took all of the control Rozanne had left not to shudder visibly.

"Jeff, what's going on?" she asked. "This isn't like you? What happened?"

Jeff came out of the daze he was in and started shouting at her "They were..." but was unable to continue because of the foam in his mouth

Rozanne quickly said, "Jeff, why don't you go and spit that out?"

He went to the garbage can by the wall and spit...and spit...and spit some more. It seemed to Rozanne to go on indefinitely. Finally, he returned. When he got back, he still had foam and snot on his face. It was incredible.

Rozanne tried again, "Jeff, what's the problem?"

Jeff began once more to shout hysterically, "They were stuffing Pixie Stix and gum and candy in my mouth, Mrs. Paxman. They were putting it in my mouth. They made me eat it."

Rozanne thought, "What's the big deal? Candy. I thought junior high kids liked candy..."

A little voice inside of her told her that something with this line of thinking wasn't right, so she told the students, "Why don't you go to lunch now? I want to think about this. I'll let you know tomorrow what I've decided to do about it. Go on now."

The students left the room, Jeff muttering to himself as he exited.

She felt like a cannon had exploded in her head. Her ears were ringing and everything was a blur. She must have gone to lunch that day, but she later—when she tried to remember it—she was unable to recall what she'd eaten and whom she'd spoken to. She must have taught the rest of her classes—but that, too, was forgotten. There was a faculty meeting that afternoon. She knew that she attended it; she always attended them. The next event she was able to recall was sitting in the district's payroll office, waiting for someone to talk to her.

A longhaired, brunette woman looked up from the desk where she was working and asked, "Are you Rozanne Paxman?"

"Yes."

The girl spun her chair around until it faced her. "You must be aware that you were overpaid by $900!"

Rozanne shook her head wearily. "No," she replied. "I didn't know this until I was informed of that at school today."

The girl looked at her inquisitively and said, "You're lucky we found out about it now. Just think how much you could have owed the school district if the overpayment had continued until the end of the school year! You'd have had a terrible time paying it off."

Rozanne could feel the tears welling up and knew that her cheeks were turning bright red. "This wasn't my fault," she said desperately. "I didn't make the mistake. Someone else had to. I don't know why everyone's acting like I did something wrong."

The girl softened her stance and said carefully. "Of course you didn't. No one is saying that. But you do have to pay it back."

Rozanne folded her hands and looked at them. "I guess I do."

"I'll tell you what," said the girl. "We'll take it out of your next check and then you'll be even. How about that?"

"You can't do that!" Rozanne cried. "How will I pay our rent? Our rent is more than a thousand dollars and I pay it out of my check! I've got to be able to pay my rent!"

"Oh, all right," the girl relented. "Then we'll take it out over two months—November and December. Then you'll have it all paid back by the end of the year."

"There's no other way to do this?" Rozanne pleaded.

"No. It has to be paid back by the end of the calendar year," stated the girl firmly.

Rozanne looked at her for a while and then mumbled, "There goes Christmas."

She jumped up from the chair she was sitting in, ran quickly from the building, and got into her minivan as fast as possible. She raced out of the parking lot and barreled up the road towards their home. As she drove, she thought wildly, "I've got lots of insurance. I even have $250,000 worth of accidental death insurance. If I roll the van and kill myself, Gary would have plenty of money to get going again and take care of the kids. I can't stand this. I can't face my life anymore. I just want to disappear."

Rozanne knew that her thoughts weren't right, but she couldn't stop them from coming, so she just concentrated on getting home. "You can do it, you can do it," she repeated to herself, over and over. When she got there, she went straight to her bedroom, crashed on her waterbed, and stared up at the ceiling. She was trying to just zone out—she didn't want to think anymore. She wanted to disappear...

"Mom. Mom. MMMOOOOOMMMM! Where are you? Has anybody see her?"

"She's in her bedroom, I think," came the reply.

Rozanne put a pillow over her head.

"Hey, Mom! What are you doing? MOM...I need to talk to you.... MOOOMMM!"

Rozanne came out from under the pillow. Two of her four children were standing by the side of the bed.

"What do you need?"

The boy looked at her impatiently. "My state report is due at school tomorrow. I need you to do it for me."

"I won't do it for you." Rozanne replied. "I can help you with it, though."

"No, Mom," he whined. "I need you to do it for me. I can't do it."

Rozanne started to breathe heavily and said, "Sure you can. It may be hard for you, but you can do it."

He stamped his foot. "No, I can't!" he yelled. "I can't do anything. I haven't learned anything in my whole life!"

Rozanne looked at him for a moment. She didn't know how to respond. Finally she blurted out, "Oh, grow up!"

Jumping off the bed, she walked quickly down the hall. Rozanne didn't know where she was going, but she wanted to get there...now! She spotted the coat closet, opened the door, sat down inside, and closed the door quietly. She didn't want them to know where she was.

She felt the heavy winter coats around her face and head. She felt safer now. As she sat there, memories began streaming through her consciousness...She remembered something that terrified her...And it was important...

Jeff Parker was a diabetic, and he had one of the most difficult cases she'd ever seen. Everyone knew about it, especially the students in that class. The 5th period choir class was right before lunch. This was the time of day when Jeff had the most trouble with his sugar level. Several times a week he would ask for permission to leave the room to check his blood levels. Just as often, he would have to be excused early to go to lunch. Even on days when he didn't go to lunch early, Rozanne would spot him sitting in his seat looking dazed. It was obviously difficult for that poor boy and those kids knew it.

They knew he was a diabetic.

They were trying to harm him!

They choose the very moment when she was behind the piano, because they knew she couldn't watch them as she read the music...and they'd put Pixie Stix (of all things!) in that boy's mouth. Pixie Stix is sort of like Jell-O...All *sugar...It would dissolve in his mouth almost instantly. That's why Jeff was spitting! Oh, it all made sense now...*

"Oh no! What will I do about this?" she thought wildly. "I can't stop it from happening. There are too many of them. I have to play the piano. I can't watch them all. I can't guarantee that boy's parents tomorrow that he'll be any safer in the room than he was today. It won't do any good to send the offenders to the office—they won't do anything. What will I do? I just want to die. I want to die. I can't do this anymore."

She began sobbing. Everything was hopeless. She was stuck. She couldn't quit. She couldn't stay.

She couldn't stand to stay.

She just wanted to die—to disappear into a dark abyss where everyone would just leave her alone.

She could hear her husband as he entered the house.

She heard him say, "Where's your mother?"

Julianne was crying. "Mommy's gone. I can't find her. I've looked everywhere."

Rozanne kept crying...She wanted to die...

She heard Gary looking for her, calling her name.

She couldn't answer...She kept crying...She just wanted to disappear...

The closet door opened. It was Gary. He looked scared when he saw her. He knelt down by her and whispered, "What's wrong?"

"I'm sick, Gary. I'm sick. I want to die. I just want to die. I can't do it anymore. I can't do it. I want to die. I'm sorry, sorry...Sorry..."

He knelt there a while, holding her. Then he got up and closed the closet door.

She heard him talking to someone, "Margaret, I don't know what to do...What? Are you sure? Okay" He hung up the phone.

The darkness of the closet closed in on her. The air became stale. The coats seemed heavier. Jeff's face flashed in her mind tormenting her. She couldn't keep him safe tomorrow. She couldn't keep any of them safe tomorrow.

She wanted to die. She wanted to die.

The phone rang. "Hello. He does? I don't know, I don't know...I can't tell her that. Will you tell her? All right."

The closet door opened and Gary handed her the telephone. "Rozanne, Margaret wants to talk to you."

"Margaret?" she whispered. "All right...Hello?"

"Rozanne, you need some help."

Rozanne began crying again. "I know...I know...I want to die, Margaret."

"I want you to agree to go to the hospital, Rozanne. It's a good one," Margaret assured. "I wouldn't send you to a bad one. I've talked to Dr. Beall, my partner—he's the Ph.D. for our office—and he agrees. You need to go to the hospital. Will you go?"

Rozanne waited.

The only sound she heard was the sound of sniffling.

She realized it was her own sniffling she heard.

She saw Jeff's face again and felt the panic well up in her soul. "Okay," she said, relinquishing her last shred of control.

Rozanne handed the phone back to Gary through the opening of the door and he closed it again. In a few minutes he re-opened the door, sat down beside her, took her in his arms and shut the closet door again.

"I'm sorry, Rozanne," he said. "I didn't realize how bad it was for you. I knew you were having problems, I guess, but I didn't know how much you were suffering. I was afraid to tell you about the hospital. I asked Margaret to tell you. I was afraid you'd get mad at me. I don't want to hurt you."

"I'm not mad, Gary," she answered. "I feel kind of relieved. I felt so afraid. I wanted to die and I was afraid I'd actually do it. It started to look like the only way out."

They sat in silence for a while before Gary said, "Rozanne, would you let me give you a blessing?"

"Yes."

He helped her out of the closet and led her back into their bedroom. He found a chair, and sat her gently down in the seat and began to speak...

She felt calmer. He got her a suitcase and she packed it. She kissed her children goodbye, and they left.

As he drove to the hospital Gary said, "I feel better now. I was afraid it wasn't the right thing to do...to take you to a hospital like this. But the influence of the spirit was so strong while I was giving you the blessing. Everything is going to work out."

Rozanne looked out the side window of the van at the images as they flashed by. She said, "I know what you mean. I don't know how, but it *will work out*. I'm sorry about the kids, though. You'll have to deal with all of that."

"Don't you worry," he assured her. "I'll take care of everything. Is there anyone you want me to call?"

Rozanne looked back over at him. "Don't call our folks. I don't want them to know. I'm afraid they'll be hurt by it. You could call my brother, though...and the Bishop and Relief Society President. I wouldn't mind them knowing. I'd like to see the Bishop as soon as I can."

Rozanne put her hands over her eyes. "But no one else, okay? This is so embarrassing. People don't understand this kind of a thing. You hear them making jokes about "losing it" and "landing in the nut house." I know I used to. Now I'm on my way to the "nut house." What a come down. Just tell the district, for now, that I'm very sick and have gone to the hospital. Tell them you'll call them as soon as you know more. It's true, you know, and it won't hurt them to think it is a regular hospital, for now. Could you do that? They'll have to know first thing in the morning so that they can arrange for a substitute."

"No problem. I'll handle everything."

When they got to the hospital, they were given papers to fill out and sign. Rozanne was worried about the insurance. She knew that their policy was tricky. She knew they needed to get a pre-authorization. The gentleman that checked her in tried to call her company, but no one answered; it was too late. He assured her, "Please don't worry about this. We've had many patients with *this same insurance policy. I'm sure you'll be fine. I'll call first thing in the morning, myself, and make sure you are authorized. I'll let you know. If you don't hear from me by noon tomorrow, you'll know that everything went well."*

"Are you sure?" she worried. "We just can't get stuck with a big bill! Not now! I couldn't stand it! How could we pay? Are you sure?"

He patted her hand. "Rozanne, really... I'm sure everything will be fine."

After they had signed the paperwork, Gary kissed her goodbye, and the man who checked her into the hospital took her back to the wing she would be staying in. She was given a brief physical by a staff member and was taken to her room. By then, she was so exhausted that she fell into a deep slumber.

"Rozanne, I think that's enough for today," said Dr. Beall. "I can see what we need to work on, but I'd like to leave it until I see you tomorrow. I've got to get back to my office. Here's my card. It has my office number as well as my pager number. If you need me, please, call the pager number. I'll get right back to you. Do you have any questions for me?"

"Not now," she replied. "I'm just trying to get through the day."

"I can certainly understand that," he said. "Oh, do you happen to have a journal?"

"I have an old one that I haven't used for years at home," she answered.

Dr. Beall smiled at her. "I'll bring you a new one. I'd like you to write down any thoughts and feelings you may have so we can talk about them. Could you do that for me?

Rozanne yawned. Telling her story had exhausted her. "I think so," she replied. "Only they won't let me have any "sharps" because I'm on red. Could you talk to them about letting me use a pen or pencil?"

"Yes. I'll have them give you one—and some paper, too. That way you can start writing today, even though you don't have your journal yet. Do you still feel you need to die?"

Rozanne thought about that. She could still see Jeff's face haunting her in her mind, but she felt so very debilitated that she knew she couldn't get the energy together to hurt herself. "No," she answered him at last. "Not really...I'm too tired."

"Good." he said. "I'll talk to them about putting you on yellow. Do you feel all right about that?"

"Yes."

Dr. Beall scrutinized her face for a moment before he continued, "Will you promise me something? Promise me that if you start feeling suicidal, you'll talk to someone about it."

The memory of her night in the closet washed over her. "I think I can do that," she said. "Okay, I promise."

"Good." he said, standing. "I'll see you tomorrow then. Remember—call me if you need me."

"I will," she promised.

When Rozanne got back into the group room, Rhaun was leading the group. She tried to sneak into the room so as to be as unnoticeable as possible. Rhaun was making an issues chart on a white-board for the group. The list read, *"Anger, Abuse, Control."*

"Come on, guys. What else do you want to talk about today?" he encouraged.

"I want to talk about abuse," said Macie. "Abuse by others. Abuse of others. Abuse of yourself. Abuse of food. Abuse."

Gloria interjected, "Macie. We know that. I wouldn't mind about talking about it, too."

"But we've talked about it almost everyday," said Heather. "I think we should talk about something else."

"What about you, Andy? What would you like to talk about?" asked Rhaun.

Andy looked up from his shoes. "I don't know. I guess, anything everyone else wants to talk about."

"Come on." Rhaun encouraged. "You must have an opinion."

Andy looked around the room at the faces of the other patients. "Well…I think maybe we could talk about anger."

"Yes, anger," said Gloria. "Anger's good. I mean, I get so mad at my mom, sometimes. I think we should talk about anger."

"What about you Heather?" Rhaun asked.

Heather shrugged her shoulders and put down her colored pencil. "Okay…Anger."

Rhaun turned and looked at Rozanne. "Is that all right with you. Rozanne?"

Rozanne started with surprise. She didn't know she was included in this decision. She replied, "Sure. Why not?"

"Tawny. Tawny!." Rhaun said loudly to the figure on the couch. "Do you want to talk about anger?" There was no reply from the love seat, so he continued, "Anger is it, then. Who wants to start?"

Heather said, "I will. It was my idea to talk about something besides abuse today. I think that almost everyone here knows that I have a reason to be angry."

Heather stopped her narration and looked out of the window. The group waited. When she was ready, she continued, "My kids…my kids were…murdered by our best friend. He's still free. We can't get anyone to do anything about it…The police blew the case so bad…They lost important evidence, but everyone seems to know that he did it."

Heather pounded her fist on the table, her voice rising in pitch as she continued. "I just can't understand how this could happen. I feel so angry about it. So angry at him…Sometimes, I just want to kill him myself. I've spent the last five years trying—trying so hard—to bring him to justice. I think about it all of the time…I've talked to everyone…the police department…the County District Attorney…the State Attorney…I've tried to get the story told in the newspapers. I've spent thousands of dollars hiring my own private detective to get enough evidence to prove that the guy did it. Nothing I do seems to help. I'm filled with so much anger that, sometimes, I think I'm going to explode!"

Heather looked around the room. Everyone was nodding in sympathy. "My other kids are suffering because of this, too. I just can't seem to get on with my life. I get so depressed that I just want to kill myself to go and be with them, but I need to be here with my other children. My husband killed himself two years ago because he couldn't handle it anymore. This makes me angry, too. Angry with the guy who killed our kids. Angry with my husband for leaving me here to deal with all of this by myself…Angry at the situation…Angry at life…just plain angry…"

As the group listened to Heather's pain, they became more and more somber. When Heather was finished, everyone sat quietly in their seats, studying the carpet like they had suddenly discovered it was made out of gold fibers.

After a while Rhaun said, "Heather, I think we all can understand why you are so angry. Unfortunately, your anger isn't hurting your children's murderer; it's hurting you. We've talked before about trying to find you an outlet that will help you deal with all of the pain you feel. Do you have any ideas?"

Heather buried her head in her arms on the table. "Sometimes I think I'd just like to hit him over and over until the pain goes away."

Macie sat straight up and exclaimed, "Yeah! Oh, oh, oh! I've got an idea. How about if the hospital gets us a punching bag or a punching dummy and we all can take turns hitting it?" "Macie, you may be on to something," said Heather, lifting her head again. "I think I'd like to have a chance to just punch something out until I get so tired that I can't stand it. Maybe it would help. How about it, Rhaun, could you do it?"

Rhaun shook his head. "I don't think that the hospital has the money for it. Besides, where would we put it?"

Colby suddenly flipped around in his seat and burst out, "I've got it! What if we bring in one of our mattresses and put it up against the wall. Then we could hit it and hit it! What do you think, Heather?"

Heather looked up with him with shining eyes. "Great idea, Colby! Could we do it, Rhaun?"

Rhaun considered the idea. "I think that it might work. I'll tell you what, I'll ask around this afternoon and find out if it would be allowed. If it is, we'll do it tomorrow, all right?"

"Great!" yelled Macie, bouncing in her seat. "Oh, I know what I'm going to do. I'm going to pretend it's my husband!" Suddenly, she stopped bouncing and looked down at her lap. "Oh, maybe not. You know, we're just newlyweds," she said. Looking up at Rhaun she continued, "He loves me, really he does. He's just too busy to come to see me."

This sudden change of attitude annoyed Heather. Turning to face Macie, she snarled, "Girl, when are you going to wake up and smell the coffee? I've been watching you here all of this time and you don't seem to get it. You've been in and out of here for six weeks and he's only come here once. He never calls you. He spends your money. Macie, you've got to get this thing figured out."

Macie met Heather's gaze. "Maybe you're right...Maybe I *will* pretend that mattress is Lou. I'll think about it tonight," she said nervously.

Rhaun looked over at Rozanne and said, "How about you? Do you have anyone you are angry at?"

"Me?" Rozanne yelped. "No, I'm just depressed, that's all. I'll be all right. Besides, I couldn't do it. I was always one of those kids who felt guilty when the teacher yelled at the class for misbehaving, even though I knew that I didn't have any part of it. Getting mad like that would make me feel too guilty."

"Guilty, huh? Sounds to me like we have something to work on with you," said Rhaun.

This made Rozanne squirm inside. She didn't know if she like this new development.

Rhaun continued, "Can't you think of a time when you got angry...really angry?"

Yes." Rozanne replied. "I can think of a time. But I just feel so guilty when I get angry that I don't like to think about it."

"Experiencing the emotion called anger is not the problem, Rozanne," Rhaun said. "It's the behaviors associated with anger that get people into trouble. It's important that you recognize anger when you feel it so that you can learn better ways of dealing with the feelings. If you don't, anger can go underground and cause you a lot of trouble."

Rhaun then turned his attention to the figure on the couch. "Tawny...Tawny...Do you have anything to be upset about?" asked Rhaun.

Tawny remained motionless on the couch.

"Come on, Tawny. You've got to start participating if you're ever going to go home," coaxed Rhaun.

Tawny moved her head so slightly that it was barely perceptible. In a tiny voice she whispered, "I want to go home."

"What? I don't think I heard you," teased Rhaun.

"I want to go home." This time it was slightly louder.

"Still can't hear you, Tawny," he pestered.

Even louder it came again, "I want to go home. I want to see my son."

Rhaun decided to see how much provoking Tawny would take before she'd act. "Oh, so you want to go home, huh?" he laughed. "You sure don't act like it.

Tawny sat up—looked at Rhaun—and said in a firm voice, "I want to go home. Today...If they don't let me go home, I'm going to run away." After making this speech Tawny settled back down on the couch in her former position—this time with her back pointed at Rhaun.

Rhaun stared at her posterior for a moment. Then, looking at his watch, he said, "I guess that's it for today gang. I'll check into the mattress thing and see all of you tomorrow."

"Hey, Rozanne! I just heard that you're on yellow now. You can come down to the cafeteria with us for lunch," bubbled Lizbeth. "You want to go and sit by me?"

"Sure."

"Good!" Lizbeth exclaimed. "Look, I've got to go down to my room for a minute. I'll see you in a few."

Lizbeth tore off down the hall and left Rozanne standing by the nurses' window alone. She wasn't alone for long because Macie spotted her and yelled out from the day room, "Hey, Rozanne. Come here a sec, will ya?"

Rozanne answered her request by walking into the day room and sitting down in a chair that faced the television. She turned it on and flipped the channels with the remote control in an effort to find something that would take her mind away.

"I hear you are going down to the cafeteria for lunch today," stated Macie.

"I think so," Rozanne replied, continuing to channel surf.

Macie got up from the couch where she was planted and stood between Rozanne and the television. "Would you do me a favor?" she asked innocently. "Would you bring me back a pop? They don't bring us pops in here for lunch and I'd really like one."

Rozanne looked at her for a moment. "Okay," she relented, uncomfortable with the request, but unable to make herself say no. "I'll see what I can do."

Suddenly they heard Lizbeth and Heather's voices in the hall. Macie rushed back to her seat and grabbed a magazine, thrusting it in front of her face. Heather noticed this as she entered the room, but said nothing. Instead she wanted to ask Rozanne a question. "Do you have any kids?"

"Yes. I have four of them."

Heather contemplated that before she continued her interrogation. "How old are they?" she asked.

"17, 12, 8 and 6…Three boys and a girl. The youngest is the only girl," answered Rozanne.

"I thought so. You look like you might be a mom."

"How many kids do you have?" Rozanne asked.

"Three boys and two girls. The oldest two, a boy and a girl, were the ones that were murdered. Now I just have the youngest three."

"Where are they now?" questioned Lizbeth.

Heather got a strained look on her face. "My mom and dad are taking care of them for me," she answered. "My parents don't understand me being here. They think I should be over it by now. Just toughen up, I guess. Besides, I don't have any insurance. My fight for justice has taken so much of my time that I couldn't work. I guess I'll be paying for this for the rest of my life, but if I don't get the help I need I'm afraid that my kids won't have even one parent left. So I am here despite my folks objections."

Heather sighed, "My parents are prominent in the community. I think that they are afraid of how others will see it…having a daughter in the psyche ward. They're from that old school of people that feel that only seriously deranged people ever go to this kind of hospital."

She walked over to the round table and sat down next to Rozanne. "But I just couldn't do it by myself," she continued. "I knew that if I didn't come back here—yes, I've been here before—I'd be dead, too. So here I am. I miss my kids, though. They'll be coming to see me on Halloween and I want to see them in their costumes. You'll get to see them then. Do you want to see a picture?"

Heather handed Rozanne a photograph of two cute children, about the ages of seven and nine years of age. They both had thick, dark hair and beautiful, big brown eyes. The older boy had his arm wrapped casually around his younger sister and both children were grinning at the camera. "These are my kids that were murdered," Heather said. "This picture was taken about three months before it happened. The boy was named Bobby and the girl was Lorie."

"They're beautiful children," said Rozanne.

"Thanks," Heather said as she studied the picture herself briefly before passing another photo to Rozanne. It was of two boys and a little girl, all with the same beautiful eyes, but with varied shades of hair, ranging from dark blond to chestnut brown. "These are the kids that I still have. Jessica, the little one, was born shortly after it happened. The other two, Adam and Rusty, were just little at the time."

Lizbeth, who had been eavesdropping, said, "Heather, I don't know how you've stood it. If anything happened to my kids, I think I'd go out of my mind."

Heather laughed. "Lizbeth, doesn't it occur to you that we *are* out of our minds. Look at where we are."

Mark appeared in the doorway. "Lizbeth…Rozanne…Are you ready to go?"

They all walked down the hallway to be joined at the double-doors by Colby, Gloria, and Andy…Still no Laura, Rozanne noticed. After buzzing the group through the security checkpoints, they all walked down the long halls to the cafeteria. Colby and Gloria walked ahead, chattering as they went.

Lizbeth busied herself by pointing out interesting facts about the hospital, warning her about food that she should be wary of, and telling her about her current boyfriend. "He's a cutie. He's helping my mom take care of my kids right now. My "ex" is nowhere to be found. I'm pretty lucky this time. I think I finally found a good guy. You'll see him. He comes over here with my mom and kids every night. Hopefully, I'll be out of here soon, though."

Lizbeth pulled at Rozanne's arm. "Look, here we are. I'll show you what you've got to do…Get a tray…Here's the silverware. I usually get the salads—they're pretty good." Lizbeth pulled a face. "Oh, yuck…look…They've made stuffed green peppers today."

"I like them," said Rozanne.

Lizbeth looked back at her. "Good for you…I guess I'll just have to eat extra stuff. Here's the pop machine. You can have as much as you want…just pour your own…"

Rozanne filled up two cups with Sprite, put on lids and got two straws. She'd take one back to Macie when they were finished.

Lizbeth continued her oration. "…They usually have ice cream. I get it at the end of the meal. That's where you put your plate and silverware when you are finished…" She continued prattling like this the entire time they were in the cafeteria. Rozanne was relieved that to hear Lizbeth's voice because she wouldn't have to talk much. She was able to listen and study the other people around the table while she ate.

Colby seemed to be what would be considered a typical "gang" type kid. Because patients weren't allowed to have belts, ties or cords, his baggy jeans kept sliding down every time he moved or walked. This forced him to constantly hold up his pants, for fear of losing them. He didn't say too much about himself, but laughed at the comments other people made.

Colby liked to eat. He had two big plates piled high with food and was downing his meal with relish. The few, but rare, comments he made about himself led Rozanne to understand that he had been in trouble with the law on a regular basis. He had managed to get away with it while he was underage, but suddenly he was eighteen, and as a legal adult, the rules had changed. Apparently, his lawyer had worked out a deal with the judge. It was decided that if Colby went into a substance abuse treatment program for thirty days, he wouldn't have to serve time in the state penitentiary. Instead, he would go on probation while continuing his therapy in the day program.

Andy came from a large family that enjoyed drinking beer after work and at every family gathering. Unfortunately, he couldn't control his drinking and had turned into an alcoholic. He'd been in a treatment program before, but had slipped back into his old habits soon after being released.

She couldn't quite get a grip on Gloria. She seemed nice enough. She didn't seem very depressed. However, she seemed to be laboring under the unfortunate opinion that she was stupid because her parents had always told her that she was "retarded." Rozanne couldn't help but think that what Gloria needed most was someone to believe in her.

Mark sat with the group as they ate and conversed easily with them. This seemed to be the norm for staff, because the members of the group seemed so comfortable with him. He kidded Gloria, joked with Colby, offered a few tips of advice to Lizbeth and talked about electronics with Andy. He seemed at ease with Rozanne's silence and would occasionally offer a nod of the head towards her to let her know that he was aware of her. He understood her need for taking her time getting into the swing of things. At the conclusion of the meal, Mark stood up signaling to the group that it was time for them to go.

After lunch, everyone went his or her own way upon getting back to the floor. They had some free time until the next group started at 1:30. Rozanne was unsure what to do so she went back to the day room, watched some television, and flipped through a few of the magazines that were there. Nothing seemed to interest her much though, and pretty soon she found that she was pacing around the room until a voice caught her attention.

It was Macie. She was out in the hall on the telephone. "When are you going to come down here?" Macie demanded. "No…No. You can't cash that check. That's my benefit check. I need that to pay the rent…No…I already told you that I wouldn't let you do that. Look, I need to know if you are going to come down here tomorrow night, like you promised me. Are you coming or not? You better…I need you to come…It's lonely here."

Rozanne felt inexplicably annoyed by what she heard so she walked across the hall and entered the group room.

Heather was at the table coloring again with Gloria. Gloria called, "Hey, Rozanne. Why don't you come and color with us?"

As she sat, she noticed that they were coloring, quite seriously, prints chosen from the large selection stacked around the table. Rozanne began shuffling through the piles of various copies of coloring book pages, geometric shapes, mazes, and craft patterns. Gloria was toiling on a page from a child's coloring book and Heather was working on a black and red geometric pattern with tiny squares. She was so engrossed in her work that, for a moment, she didn't even seem aware that Rozanne had sat down right next to her.

"Gosh, I don't think I've colored for more than twenty years," Rozanne exclaimed.

The sound of Rozanne's voice broke Heather's concentration and she looked up from the page, "Go ahead," she said. "It's amazing how it makes you feel better. Look at all of the sheets I've colored in the last couple of days."

She showed Rozanne eight pages of varying topics that were beautifully done. Heather admired her work briefly. "I'm going to put them on the walls in my room. I think I'll be here for a while, so I want to make it feel more like it's my own space. Some of the pictures I give to my children when they come to see me. They like the idea that mom is coloring pictures for them."

Rozanne selected a view of a flying unicorn gliding over the San Francisco Bay and went to work. It did seem to have the desired effect and she soon found herself relaxing. She'd always loved color…any color…especially combinations of color. There was a time that the colors of the world seemed to glisten around her…everything was so bright and beautiful. Once, when she was visiting her grandfather, she saw a double rainbow and the sight was so beautiful that she cried. She suddenly realized that colors had faded for her over the past several years—just like someone had slowly turned a dimmer switch to the left—so slowly that she hadn't realized that it was happening. Where had the colors gone and why did everything seem so gray now?

A petite blond-haired woman in her early fifties walked purposely into the room and interrupted them. "Time for group, gang. Why don't you come on over here and sit down."

Rozanne obediently got up and moved over to the corner of the long leather couch. It was out of the line of action and she hoped that she'd go unnoticed. She had no such luck because immediately, the woman turned sharply and faced her. "You're new here. What's your name?"

"Rozanne."

"Hi, Rozanne. I'm Carol Swanson. I lead the chemical dependency group. Everyone has to come, even if that isn't the reason you're here. You'll find that you'll hear things that will help you, if you'll be open minded."

Colby and Lizbeth burst into the room and threw themselves down onto two of the empty chairs at the table by Heather and Gloria, who were still coloring intently. They immediately began whispering and giggling to each other as they started to work on projects of their own. Andy quietly followed. As he took a seat on the love seat facing Rozanne, he smiled a small, hopeful smile at her. Tawny shuffled in next and made a beeline to the remaining long couch, where she took up residence in her accustomed fetal position.

"Where's Macie?" asked Carol.

"The last time I saw her, she was bugging staff about wanting to talk to her doctor," said Lizbeth. "She's insisting that she's being starved to death."

"I am being starved to death!" Macie yelled as she strutted into the room. "I can't stand it, I tell you. I haven't had enough to eat in three days. It's not fair...Everybody else gets to go to the cafeteria.... Everybody else gets to drink pop. Why did they have to take my pop away from me? It was just a little cup."

"How did you get it, Macie?" asked Carol. "You're not supposed to drink pop."

"I'm not telling." Macie put her hands defiantly on her hips and glared at Carol briefly before tossing her head and striding over to take a seat on the couch next to Rozanne. Rozanne felt her face becoming flushed. "What have I done now?" she thought.

Heather saw Rozanne's expression and took action. "What are we going to do today?" she asked Carol. "I hope we are going to talk about something new. Sometimes it seems like we just go around and around in these groups."

Rozanne glanced over at Heather gratefully and Heather winked in reply.

"Well, what do you think we should talk about?" Carol asked.

"I was hoping we could talk about coping skills."

"I guess that's all right," responded Carol. "What do the rest of you think?"

"That sounds great to me," agreed Andy.

Carol looked at Andy inquisitively. "I don't think I've met you yet."

Andy reached up from the loveseat at shook her hand. "I'm Andy. I just came in last night. This is the second time around for me. Coping skills are probably what I need the most.

"What about you, Rozanne?" Carol asked. "What do you do to cope?

"Me?" asked Rozanne in surprise.

Carol nodded firmly. "Yes, you."

Rozanne pulled her knees up to her chest and hugged them. "You know that I'm here for depression, don't you?" she replied. She didn't know why Carol was focusing on her. She had imagined that she could just sit and listen during this group.

Carol was unmoved. "I know that. You felt suicidal, right?"

Rozanne nodded.

"There had to be something that you were doing before last night to help you cope. What did you spend your time doing"

Rozanne contemplated her answer. Just what had she been doing besides teaching school? Then she remembered. "TV," she said. "I watched TV...Lots and lots and lots of TV. When I'm watching TV I don't have to think about anything at all. I think TV is my "drug" of choice. I just lie there and zone out."

Colby and Lizbeth began giggling.

"What's so funny, Colby?" Carol inquired.

Colby shrugged innocently as he continued coloring. "Nothing…nothing at all…"

Heather interjected, "So then, Colby…Why don't you tell us how *you* cope with problems?"

"Me," he laughed. "I ain't got no problems that twenty-three more days in this joint won't cure. I'll be out of here and that will be that. Then I'm going to cope by going home and finding my buddies and we'll just pick right up where we left off."

Carol stared long and hard at Colby's back before she said, "That may be so, Colby. But the time is coming that you will have to finally face whatever you are running so hard to get away from. You're just a kid. I wish you could care about yourself just a little. Maybe you'd look around you at the people coming in and out of here and see what drugs and alcohol has brought them to and avoid that scene for yourself."

"Amen." Lizbeth whispered. Lifting her head from her coloring she looked over at Colby. "My dad was heavy into that whole thing, Colby. He took off when I was just a kid. My mom tried to do the best she could by us kids, but it was tough. She worked three jobs raising us and I got married when I was seventeen just to get out of the house. Then after having three kids of my own and a husband who ran around on me, I finally got the guts to get out of that bad situation and try to move forward myself. He was a drunk, too, you know. But then it all came crashing down on me one day…"

Lizbeth picked up a different colored pencil and scribbled angrily as she continued talking. "I was at work—I work for the telephone company as an operator—and a customer called and wanted to get some help calling Japan. I just suddenly started yelling and crying and carrying on…for no reason, really. I guess it just got to me—the whole thing. I was suddenly my mom and I was going to have to work all of those jobs because I got hooked up with someone like you who only could think of the next time that he was going to get high. I just couldn't do it. I wanted out of there. I wanted out of my life."

Lizbeth stopped coloring and looked out of the window. "My boss could tell that something was seriously wrong. He took me into his office and got me a soda and told me he was going to call our insurance company and get me some help. He made some calls and convinced me I needed to come here…He was right—I didn't know it then and I didn't know it this morning—but he was right."

Lizbeth turned her chair slightly and looked at Carol. "Carol, I need to learn some things. I need to learn to change things around. I can't do this to my kids. I've got to break this cycle."

Colby grunted, got up, moved two chairs away from Lizbeth and began coloring his picture with vehemence.

Macie, who had been scowling during this whole interchange suddenly announced, "Well, I don't think that you have a clue. At least your mother wanted you! My mother told me when I was six years old that she wished I had never been born. She was ashamed of me. I was stupid in school and she said that she wasn't surprised a bit. She said that I was like my idiot father and that she'd been crazy to take up with him. But she was still married to the man. She still is and she acts like she likes him just fine. So, what I want to know is why she doesn't want me. What's wrong with *me*?"

Rozanne felt her stomach tighten. She'd never heard such terrible things expressed before. It made her problems seem like nothing. She had a family that loved her. She had a husband who was a worthy priesthood holder who was extremely patient and kind to her. She had four children. Most importantly, she had the knowledge of the truthfulness of the Gospel of Jesus Christ. Why hadn't it been enough? What hadn't she been able to cope? She must be doing something wrong—but what?

"What's wrong, Rozanne?" asked Carol, noticing the pained expression on Rozanne's face.

"I just feel awful," Rozanne replied. "Everyone here has such terrible problems. Mine are nothing in comparison to theirs. I feel guilty being here."

Carol's face softened as she replied, "There is obviously something you need, Rozanne, or you wouldn't be here. Work hard during your stay and I'm willing to bet that you get your answers."

After group was over Rozanne decided to go down to her room for a while. Before she made it, Gloria chased her down to talk. "Can I ask you a question?" she asked forcefully. "Are you an active member?"

"Of what?" asked Rozanne vaguely, not wanting to become involved in any more conversations for a while.

Gloria shook her head impatiently. "The church—the Mormon church. Macie says you're a member."

Rozanne gave up. She turned back and faced Gloria. "Yes," she replied. "I'm active."

"I thought so." Gloria said. "You look different than the rest of us."

Rozanne shook her head impatiently at Gloria. She'd never felt so low in her life. What on earth was Gloria talking about? "What do you mean?"

"I don't know how to explain it," Gloria said, pulling on the neck of her sweatshirt. "Maybe you've heard that I'm retarded. I only have an IQ of 90 and my mom told me I'm retarded."

Rozanne met Gloria's eyes. "You know what? I've been meaning to talk to you about that. When I studied IQ's in college, I learned that people with IQ's between 80 and 120 fall in the normal range. So you see, 90 is normal, not retarded. Where did your mother get that idea?"

"Normal?" Gloria stammered. "90 is normal?"

Rozanne nodded.

Gloria shook her head in disbelief. "Nobody has ever told me that before."

Rozanne reached out and touched Gloria's arm. "It's true. Check it out. There are lots of books on that sort of thing in libraries."

"I can't believe it," Gloria groaned. "Really? Are you sure? Why would my mom tell me that I'm retarded if I'm not?"

Rozanne sighed, "I don't know. I just don't know. Maybe she just doesn't understand what that term really means."

Gloria slunk dejectedly over to the hall wall and slid down onto the floor. She held her head and began moaning with a low, breathy tone that reminded Rozanne of a hot wind blowing through a leaky window.

Instinct took over and Rozanne got down on the floor next to Gloria and put her arms around the broken figure that was rocking back and forth in despair. She felt desperate to break the spell Gloria was under. "Why did you want to know if I'm an active Mormon?" she asked.

Gloria stopped rocking to look at Rozanne. "Did you know that I went on a mission?"

Rozanne nodded in reply. Gloria took a deep breath and went on. "A little while after I came home from my mission I went inactive. I just got so low…and then I moved around. I don't even know who my bishop is anymore. I've also let some guys take advantage of me and I've had trouble with the Word of Wisdom, you get the picture? Now I'm thinking that I need to get myself straightened out. I've been here for a while and I'm feeling better. I'll be going home in a couple of days. I was wondering if you could get me a Book of Mormon to read."

Rozanne replied, "Oh, is that all you want? Sure, I'd be happy to do that. I'll call my husband."

Gloria smiled. The crisis, for the moment, was over. "Great! I was also wondering something else. Could you help me to get a blessing? I don't talk to my parents right now and like I told you, I don't know who my bishop is. I'd really like a blessing."

"I guess so," Rozanne answered. "My bishop and husband are coming tomorrow night and I could ask them to give you one, if you'd like."

Gloria jumped up. "Would you really? Oh, that would be so great!" She scampered down the hall shouting, "Macie! Macie! I'm going to get a blessing!"

The sudden shift in Gloria's mood left Rozanne feeling breathless. She sat on the floor until she felt strong enough to continue down to her room. Once she arrived, she sat on her bed and looked around the room. No Laura…How strange…Where could she be?

Picking up her scriptures from the bedside table, she began thumbing through the pages. It seemed like a long time had gone by since she had studied them. She always meant to read them, but she couldn't seem to find the time.

Time was so slippery. She had to get up at 5:30 in the morning to get ready for work and then she had to get the kids up, make lunches and be at school by 6:45. She rarely made it home before 6:00 in the evening and then there was dinner, homework, kids, bed, and more. Then she'd either zone out in front of the TV or fall into bed, where she'd sleep fitfully the whole night.

It hadn't always been that way. Her patriarchal blessing told her how important scripture study and prayer would be to her during her life. She knew it was true, but she had a hard time disciplining herself to be regular about doing what she knew to be right.

And then there were her prayers…

She'd always prayed on her knees all during her girlhood and throughout her early years of marriage. Then Gary and Rozanne bought a king-sized waterbed that was high off of the floor. Before long, they began praying while lying in bed. After a while, she let Gary say most of the prayers because she felt that her prayers were basically bouncing off of the ceiling. She'd never been too good about praying in the morning…It always seemed that she just jumped up and ran into the day full steam ahead. She did pray in her mind off and on and it amazed her that the Lord seemed to answer those prayers.

"There's got to be more to this that I realize," she said out loud to herself. "How did I get in such a mess?"

Rozanne knelt by the bed and began, "Heavenly Father, I don't know what to say to you, but I need thy help. I'm not quite sure how I got here.

I just know that this isn't a very nice place to be in my life. Please be with me. Please forgive me. Help my family while I'm here. I'm sure the kids don't understand what's going on and they've got to be scared. Help me to find the answers I need to become well again. I say these things in the name of Jesus Christ. Amen."

She picked her scriptures up again and began aimlessly looking through the book. Then a passage in Roman's chapter one caught her eye, "Who shall separate us from the love of Christ?" she read, "Shall tribulation, or distress, or persecutions, or famine, or nakedness, or peril or sword? Nay, in all these things we are more than conquerors through him that loved us. For I am persuaded, that neither death, nor life, nor angels, nor principalities, nor powers, nor things present, nor things to come, nor heights, nor depth, nor any other creature, shall be able to separate us from the love of God, which is in Christ Jesus our Lord."

"Oh, please let it be true," she whispered desperately. "Please...let it be true."

After dinner, Gary came to visit her. He brought pictures Julianne and Andrew had drawn with "I love you, Mom" and hearts sprawled all across the sheets.

Rozanne traced the hearts with her finger. "How are they doing?" she asked him.

"They're pretty upset, but they'll be all right. I don't want you to worry about them."

"What about Halloween? I didn't get their costumes ready yet."

"I'll take care of that," he replied. "You just concentrate on getting well so you can come home. I won't be able to come here Halloween night, though. Stephen is going to stay home and pass out the candy so that I can take the little kids around trick-or-treating."

"That's okay."

Gary looked around the room. It looked different than he imagined it would. He thought that maybe it would look like the day room in "One

Flew Over the Cuckoo's Nest." They had gone to see that movie on their honeymoon, but found it so disturbing that they walked out of the theater after about a half an hour. This place looked like the break room at work. "Do you want me to bring the kids here to see you?" he asked.

"I don't know yet. Maybe I'll have a better idea tomorrow night when you come. Did you get a chance to talk to the bishop yet?"

"Yes. He's coming tomorrow night to see you. He wants to know if it's all right to tell the Relief Society President and the Compassionate Service Leader what has happened so that they can bring in some meals for the family."

Rozanne's first impulse was to refuse, but then she decided that wasn't being fair to Gary. Meals would help him. "I guess so," she told him. "I guess I can trust them. I don't want anyone to know—other than them. It's just too embarrassing. Could you ask the Relief Society President if there is some way to keep it quiet? I know…Maybe the meals could be delivered to her house—then she could take them to our house. I just don't want people to know who is getting all of those meals. People are so curious…

She was frying hamburger when the impression came that she needed to call Lucy. The longer she stirred the meat, the stronger the feeling came. She finally picked up the phone and dialed. "Hi, Lucy. It's Rozanne. This is going to sound strange, but I suddenly got the feeling I should call you and ask you if everything is all right."

The other end of the phone was silent for thirty long seconds. She could hear breathing on the other end and she knew that Lucy was still there, so she waited. Finally the reply came, "How did you know?"

"Know what?" Rozanne asked.

Lucy's voice sounded stunned. "You don't know?"

An uneasy feeling began growing inside of Rozanne. She ignored it and continued, "No…I just got the feeling that I should call."

Another long pause began. Rozanne began to feel her heart pound. Something was wrong with Lucy.

"Rozanne, can I come over to see you tomorrow?"

"Sure." she answered. She didn't know what to say next, so she waited. Soon Lucy asked, "How about ten?"

"That'll be fine," Rozanne replied.

After she hung up the phone, she began to worry. Lucy was her friend, although they weren't as close as she'd like them to be. Lucy was one of the other good musicians in the ward and she played the piano for the choir that Rozanne led. Lucy had five children—two boys and three girls—and a very nice husband. Rozanne had never suspected that something was wrong at their house. What on earth was going on?

The next morning she hurried and cleaned her house totally before Lucy came. She didn't want Lucy to think that she couldn't take care of her home. For some reason, she made a special point to mop the kitchen floor.

At 10:00, Lucy silently entered Rozanne's living room. She sat nervously on the couch, fiddling with the throw pillows as she spoke. "Rozanne, I'm in terrible trouble. I began having flashbacks about six months ago of being sexually abused by my father when I was a little girl. I came from an active family and so when I got about fourteen, I went to my bishop. Unfortunately, my bishop didn't believe me. I guess I must have gone out of my mind, because I felt like I had no one that I could trust."

Lucy continued her tale, not noticing the pained expression crossing Rozanne's face. "I don't remember the next few years. I was finally able to get out of there and go away to college. Somehow I managed to make myself forget all about it. I didn't remember what happened at all. I married Dave, had the kids and figured everything was fine. I just knew that for some unknown reason, I didn't like going home to visit. Last summer, when we were visiting my parents, I saw my youngest girl sitting on my father's lap and it began coming back to me. I was horrified! I made up some excuse to come back early so no one would know what was going on."

Lucy sighed and pulled absentmindedly at a stray lock of hair. "That was the beginning of a long nightmare that I can't seem to wake up from. I've totally fallen apart at home. Everything is in the biggest mess. No on knows how bad it is but the kids and Dave."

"I finally told Dave what was going on." *Lucy continued.* "I farmed the kids out with friends and then left him a letter at home with a key to the motel room where I was waiting. The letter told him everything. I told him in the letter that if he still wanted to be married to me he should come to the room. If he didn't come, I'd understand.

Lucy wiped her nose on her sleeve. "He came. I cried. He cried. I don't know what to do now. I'm so despondent that I don't think I can go on. I've been trying to work with a friend in town that seems to know about these things, but I think that I'm getting worse, not better. I feel that my life is worthless."

Rozanne was stunned. How could this be happening to her friend and she didn't know anything about it? How could she not be able to tell that something was seriously wrong with Lucy? How could she go to church week after week, work with Lucy at choir, and still not be able to pick up that she was so troubled? "It's a good thing that Heavenly Father knows everything," *she thought,* "because Lucy needs my help. I'm so glad I listened to that prompting!"

She swallowed and asked, "Lucy, what can I do?"

"I don't know..."

Rozanne waited. When it was obvious that Lucy wasn't going to say more, she took the initiative. "Well...how are things at your home? I mean, do you need food?"

Lucy looked up at her with tears in her eyes. "Rozanne, I'm in such bad shape that I can't even begin to tell you."

"Father, what do I do? What *can* I do?" *Rozanne prayed silently.* "Take her home," *the reply came quietly in her mind.*

Rozanne stood and said to Lucy, "Why don't we go to your house and then maybe I can tell better what to do?"

"Okay," *Lucy whispered.*

Rozanne was dismayed at the sight that met her eyes upon entering Lucy's home. It was dirty.

No, dirty wasn't the right word.

This home was filled with the kind of filth that gets children taken away from parents. There was litter in every spot imaginable…Dirty clothes were everywhere…Dirty dishes, leftover food, and even mouse droppings covered the kitchen countertops…The children's mattresses smelled of urine. Several of them were still wetting the bed at night and no one thought to change the bedding in the morning…

It hadn't always been this way. Lucy had invited Rozanne's family over several times to dinner and Rozanne had visited occasionally, although it had been quite a while. But it had been normal…clean…Rozanne thought to herself, "If she feels anything like this house looks I've got to do something about this today!"

She immediately telephoned the ward Relief Society President who rushed to join them. This kind woman organized a small group of sisters to come in and clean up the mess the next day.

At 4:30, Dave came home from work. Something about seeing other people in the middle of the filth snapped him out of the state of denial he was in and he made the decision to check Lucy into a hospital. He told Rozanne that he had found Lucy with a bottle of pills the night before—right about the same time Rozanne had made the phone call. Together they managed to find enough clean clothing of Lucy's to pack in the large, black suitcase he had used on his mission.

Before long Dave drove off with Lucy sitting in the front passenger seat staring forward with blank eyes, clutching desperately at Mr. Snow—the large white teddy bear that Dave had given her for Valentine's day that year—in her arms.

With Dave's permission, phone calls were made and places for the kids to stay were obtained. Rozanne took the two oldest children, the two boys, home with her.

The next day she and the other helpers and began attacking the filth in Lucy's home. She gathered all of the dirty clothing, took it home and washed it. It was a large mountain of dismayed cloth that took up residence in her garage as she washed, dried, and sorted it out. She discovered that the children didn't have enough clothes that fit them, so the Relief Society President worked on solving that problem.

Three days later, Dave's sister arrived from Tennessee and took charge of the family and Rozanne's close involvement in the family ended. Rozanne's help had been appreciated, but now her presence reminded the family of the desperate situation from which they were trying to distance themselves.

Six weeks later Lucy came home. She was different, so very different...

But the worst problem the family now faced was the realization that ward members had done a lot of discussing the "terrible situation" at Lucy's house during her absence. It had taken quite a few ward members to solve the problems the family had and unfortunately some of the "helpers" had loose tongues. Before long, wild stories were raging through the ward. Lucy had to face taking control of her life again and dealing with the curious looks and questions of ward members who wanted to know information that simply wasn't any of their business.

"Gary, you've got to promise me that you won't tell anyone else. You've got to promise!" Rozanne pleaded.

Gathering her into his arms he assured, "Rozanne, don't worry about it. I promise."

After the evening community group, Ramona tapped Rozanne on the arm. "Hey, Rozanne," she said. "Dr. Fielding is coming in tonight to give you a physical. He's an Internist. We like to make sure that there's nothing wrong with you physically when you come in. I'll let you know when he's ready for you. In the meantime, you need to go to the nurses' window and get your meds that Dr. Manning left for you."

"Dr. Manning?"

"Yes," Ramona continued. "He's the psychiatrist that was on call last night. Don't you remember talking to him?"

Rozanne couldn't remember for a moment, but then she recalled a tall, thin, blond man she had talked to. "Oh, yes. I think I can vaguely remember telling someone about what had happened at school."

"That's him," said Ramona. "He'll be your psychiatrist while you are here. He'll prescribe your antidepressants, sleeping medicines and anything else you need during your stay."

"What about Dr. Beall?"

Ramona frowned. "He's a psychologist. Didn't you know that? He'll treat you emotionally, but he doesn't prescribe medications."

Rozanne didn't know that. She had only met Dr. Beall that morning.

She went to the window and was given two medications: Paxil (an antidepressant) and some sort of sleeping medication with a long name. Almost immediately she was called down to see Dr. Fielding.

He was a short, round man with a hairline similar to Mr. Mooney of the old Lucille Ball sitcoms. In fact, he reminded Rozanne of Mr. Mooney. "Tell me about how you've been feeling," he asked her.

"What? Besides being depressed, you mean?" she asked.

"Yes."

She considered the question for a moment. Should she give him the short version or the long version? She decided to go with the short version. She was tired.

"I have Fibromyalgia," she said. "I have been taking Sinoquin for quite a long time for the sleeping disorder, but it recently stopped working for me. My family doctor gave me some Amatriptylin to try. I don't like it. It makes me feel so groggy and out of it—sort of like I had taken a powerful decongestant. That's why I decided not to take anymore of it. I hate feeling out of it and the Amatriptylin makes my mind foggy. I want my mind working."

"You probably were just taking too much of it." Dr. Fielding-Mooney said. "Amatriptylin really is the best thing I've found to give patients with

Fibromyalgia. Can't I persuade you to give it another try? How much were you taking, anyway?"

"50 milligrams," she replied.

"How about I give you 25 milligrams?"

"Too much."

"Would you consider taking half of a 25 milligram pill?" he compromised. "Lack of sleep can increase or even cause depressive symptoms."

Rozanne thought about that. Maybe it would work and she wanted to be able to sleep better. Fibromyalgia had the effect of making her have all sorts of crazy dreams.

"The first lady needs you in her office right away!"

Rozanne looked up from her desk. She was the personal secretary to the First Lady of the United States of America. It was quite an honor and now the First Lady needed her—little old Rozanne Paxman! She hurried into the office and said, "What's up?"

The first lady looked up from the pad she was scribbling notes on desperately. "I've just had some terrible news. The President went to Wyoming on a little hunting trip—he managed to sneak away without anyone knowing—and I've just received word from the Secret Service boys that he's out there causing quite a ruckus. I need you to go out there with me and help me settle the situation."

Soon they were jetting across the country in Air Force One. "What on earth is he into now?" Rozanne thought self-righteously, as she drank the virgin Strawberry Daiquiri that the stewardess had prepared. "I don't know how she stands it!"

When they arrived in Cheyenne, a Secret Service agent drove them in a military jeep out to the countryside to steep hill. They were horrified to see the President, with only his shirt, vest, and boxers on. He was drunk as a skunk and was wildly shooting a pistol about in the air while yelling about those terrible "Enquirer Wants to Know" people. Rozanne and the First Lady got down on their stomachs in their designer business suits and began snaking up the side of the hill, trying to get to him without getting shot in the head. The First Lady kept muttering, "Oh, dear. We've got to stop him before the media finds out! We'll never live this down!"

I guess I'll try it," she told Dr. Fielding-Mooney.

He smiled triumphantly. "Good...but do me a favor...You've got to try it for at least two weeks before you'll be able to tell if it helps you. You gave up too soon before."

Dr. Fielding-Mooney then gave her a complete physical, including checking out the pressure points that Fibromyalgia patients find sensitive to confirm in his own mind that she had Fibromyalgia...She did.

"Physically, you seem fine," he told her at last. "I think that you'll find the Amatriptylin will make a difference and you'll be able to sleep better. It's important to get your rest when you are trying to fight emotional battles. Some depressed patients sleep too much...some too little...Your Fibromyalgia probably doesn't help."

"Thanks. Can I go now? I've taken the sleeping pill that Dr. Manning ordered and I feel like I am going to fall over."

Dr. Fielding-Mooney nodded as he patted her on the back. "Sure. Sleep well, Rozanne...Sleep well."

Day 2

▼

After she showered and ate her breakfast, Rozanne wandered into the day room to watch a little TV. Regis and Kathie Lee would be on and she wanted to zone out. It was easier than worrying about what was ahead of her. Regis had just started asking the home contestant the question of the day when Heather came in. "You really watch that stuff?" she said.

Rozanne was unfazed. She didn't care what anyone thought this morning. "Believe it or not, I do"

Heather sat down in the chair next to Rozanne. "Why on earth do you waste your time like that?"

Rozanne kept her eyes directed towards the television screen. Maybe Heather would go away…

But she could see through her peripheral vision that Heather was waiting for her to answer, so she finally gave in and answered the question. "I guess after a while you start getting to know them. Even if you don't like everything they say, they get familiar to you…The show is always just about the same. They argue and philosophize for about fifteen minutes.

Then the guests start coming on to hock whatever they want you to buy into. They smooze with the celebrities. It's surreal. It's so far removed from my life that it's easy to forget what I am worrying about."

"I never thought about it that way," Heather said as she, too, turned her attention to the screen. They sat in companionable silence, watching Regis and Kathie Lee bicker about the value of a new book until the next commercial break began.

"Hey Heather, what's going on with my roommate, Laura," she whispered at the break. "She never comes to group and you almost never see her around. Why doesn't she have to work the program like everybody else?"

Heather whispered back, "I don't know. That is one of the great mysteries of life around here. I've been wondering about it myself. I guess I have so much on my mind that I haven't taken the time to figure out what's going on."

Suddenly, their attention was drawn to a commotion in the hall. The voices were muffled at first, but in a matter of seconds one voice became very recognizable. It was Macie.

"You know you really bug me, don't you? All I wanted was a little syrup on my pancakes and you act like it was a federal crime—like I was breaking into Fort Knox and stealing all of the gold. What's the big deal? A little syrup won't hurt me."

"Macie, when will you get it into your head?" someone replied in an annoyed tone. "The doctor has explained it over and over to you. You have a borderline case of diabetes. You can't have sugar. You can't have candy. You can't have syrup. You need to drop some weight. You are at terrible risk right now. Dr. Manning feels that if you can start to manage your eating habits better and we help you with your lifestyle choices, maybe, just maybe, you can avoid some of the terrible consequences diabetes can bring. Macie, we are trying to help you."

"Jeez," Macie replied, "you don't have to make such a big deal out of everything. I don't see how a little bit of some good stuff now and then could possibly hurt me. I think you're all just trying to punish me. I think you're just like everybody else. You don't like me, that's all. You don't want me to be happy. f you did, you'd understand why I want to have a little syrup. I can't stand to live like this!"

Rozanne and Heather recognized the voice Macie was arguing with now. It was Ramona. The could almost hear her strengthen her physical stance in an effort to convince Macie that she was serious, as she sternly retorted, "Macie, you've just got to try to *listen*. You're a borderline diabetic. It *is* a big deal—or it will be, if you won't cooperate. You're only hurting yourself, Macie."

"I want to talk to Dr Manning! I want to see that loser right now! Do you hear me? I said, I want to see him right now!"

"Macie, settle down" Ramona calmly replied, "or you'll have to go into isolation. I'll try to get him on the phone. I'll tell him you want to see him as soon as he can find the time."

Rozanne and Heather heard thumping on the wall as Macie yelled, "That's not good enough. I want to see him right now!"

"Macie, I have to warn you for the last time."

"What? What?" snarled Macie in a tone that reminded Rozanne of some of the students in her 5th period choir. "What ya gonna do, huh? Ya gonna beat me? Ya gonna tie me up? Ya gonna put me in *isolation*? We'll see about that!"

Rozanne and Heather heard scuffling sounds in the hall, followed by running…BOOM…and CRASH! They looked at each other in amazement before running into the hall to see what had happened.

Their eyes were immediately drawn to the sight of Macie writhing about in pain on the floor by the big double doors. Apparently, she had tried to get away from Ramona. A chase had developed and Macie had unwittingly smacked into them.

Ramona stood over Macie with her hands on her hips. "Macie, I've had it with you this morning. Now you're going into isolation until you can control yourself. As soon as you're able to calm down and be reasonable, you can rejoin the group. Do you understand?"

A low groan emitted from Macie. "Yes...Just get me Dr. Manning."

"I already promised you that I would," said Ramona said. "Are you going to come with me willingly or do we have to get someone down here to escort you?"

Macie looked up at Ramona with fear in her eyes. "No! Don't do that! I'll go...I'll go..."

Heather turned to Rozanne, rolled her eyes and said, "Are you ready to go into morning group yet? It's about time."

Rozanne meekly followed Heather into the next room, but her eyes followed Macie as she was escorted into the staff area. She saw that two rooms behind the staff window were numbered one and two. Macie was led into the first room and Ramona closed the door. Macie looked out of the little vertical rectangular window above the doorknob. Rozanne's eyes met Macie's briefly before Macie turned away and disappeared inside.

"Heather," Rozanne asked, "what are those rooms inside the staff area?"

Heather tossed her head in disgust. "Isolation rooms. They only put you there if they think you may be a danger to yourself or somebody else. They aren't used very often, but Macie likes to push the limits. I'm starting to get worried about her. I'm afraid that if she doesn't start to get control of herself, she'll end up at the state psyche ward. They only send you there if they think that your problems are getting to be long term and they can't help you here anymore."

As they entered the group room, Rozanne could see that most of the patients were already assembled. Gloria was in her usual corner of the long couch with Andy at the opposite end.

Tawny was curled up in a ball on the love seat. One would assume that she was asleep, but Rozanne suspected that she wasn't. Lizbeth and Colby were coloring at the table. Everyone was there but Laura...still no Laura.

When Rozanne went to bed the night before, Laura was already asleep with her back to the door, so Rozanne couldn't see her face. She didn't even stir while Rozanne prepared herself for bed, read scriptures and said her prayer. When Ramona came to get them up this morning, Laura didn't stir and Ramona didn't insist. How strange…

Rhaun entered the room with a big grin on his face. "Hey gang! I did it! I talked to my boss and he said that we could use a mattress. Andy and Colby, will you help me drag one down from an empty room?"

It was if someone had turned on the master switch of a power cord; the group began to mutter excitedly and shift in their seats in anticipation of what was going to happened next—all of them except Rozanne and Tawny. Rozanne got a weird feeling in her stomach. The whole thing sounded questionable to her.

Macie must have sensed that something was up because, at that very moment, she wandered casually into the room and announced, "Well, I guess I've enough of that for today! I showed them, didn't I? Nothing like a little early morning commotion to stir up the blood. I told them I'm fine now, so here I am. What's going on?"

"We're going to get the mattress, Macie," announced Gloria.

Macie clapped her hands gleefully, "Oh! Oh! Oh! Really! Can I go first? Can I, Rhaun? Can I? I've been thinking about it all night and I've decided that I want to go first *sooo* bad. I want to punch that mattress out. I'm going to pretend that it's my husband and my mom and anyone that's every hurt or bugged me. Please, Rhaun, let *me* go first!"

Rhaun looked around the room, "What do all of you think about Macie going first?"

"Oh, let her," said Heather. "She'll just drive us all crazy until she gets her turn."

"Yeah, let Macie go first, Rhaun. I can't wait to see this!" laughed Colby.

Colby, Andy and Rhaun went down the hall, got a mattress off of one of the beds and soon had it leaning against one of the walls. When they had finished, Rhaun announced, "Macie, it's all yours."

Macie got up from her chair and walked over to the mattress. She poked it with her right index finger, then she softly punched it with her fist.

Colby yelled, "Is that the best you can do?"

She spun around and glared at him. Then she faced the mattress and started backing away from it. She reminded Rozanne of a bull facing a matador. Macie almost seemed to paw at the floor. Suddenly, to the group's surprise, she started running full steam towards the mattress. The impact of her collision was so great that it caused her large frame to bounce off of the mattress and she landed sprawled out on the floor.

The room was immediately filled with hysterical laughter. They all laughed and laughed until tears ran from their eyes—all of them except Macie and Heather. Macie remained in place looking at the mattress with a shocked look on her face. Finally, she rolled over and awkwardly climbed back to her feet. The rest of the patients tried to get control of themselves as she stood, but it was to no avail when Macie triumphantly announced, "Well, I guess I showed you!"

The mood shifted when Heather got up and walked over to face her enemy. She rolled up her right sleeve, made a fist, clenching her hand until the veins popped out on the back of it. She took a big breath, blew it out, and took another big breath—holding it momentarily. Her eyes squinted as she imagined the mattress taking on the form of her children's murderer. When she started punching, it was with vehemence. "I hate you. I hate you," she snarled. "I hate you, you filthy murderer."

Heather gasped for air. "I know what you did," she moaned, "I've always known what you did. You and that lousy wife of yours…You started that fire because you beat my boy. I saw him that night, his broken body lying on that cold, steel gurney in the children's hospital. I saw his bruised up face. I knew what you'd done. No fire did that. You did it. You started that fire because you were too big of a coward to face us after you beat my boy. Then you left my kids in that room asleep and you walked out of the house like there was nothing wrong. Your wife even took the time to get her purse! There she was, standing on the lawn with her purse like she was going to a party or something when the fire department came. All the time you knew that my kids were dying inside your house. I hate you...I hate you...I hate you..."

When Heather's anger was spent, she collapsed on the floor in a heap, panting for air. She had pounded the mattress so violently that her hair clip had fallen out and she was in a state of total disarray. The room experienced the kind of hush that you feel in a mortuary—a cold but reverent still that makes a mourner feel the air down to the depths of their lungs. No one knew what to say—not even Rhaun. They all just sat there, afraid to move. Rozanne was terrified of what would happen next.

Heather was the one finally who broke the terrible spell. She simply got up and went back to her chair. Bending forward, she twisted her long, black hair until it was in a tight, shiny roll. Then, as she sat back in her seat, she arranged it carefully into the large white butterfly clip that had been holding it. She looked over at Rozanne and asked in a strained voice, "Why don't I feel better, Rozanne...Why?"

Rozanne met Heather's sad gaze. "Heather," she moaned, "if I had the answer to your question maybe, just maybe, I wouldn't be here."

Rozanne wandered out in the hall, after the group meeting had concluded, to be met by Dr. Beall and a small, thin gray-haired woman. "Hi, Rozanne," he said. "This is Marjorie West, the hospital administrator. She needs to talk to you. Why don't you come in here?"

Dr. Beall led Rozanne and Marjorie into the small room they had used the day before. After they were seated he began, "Rozanne, the hospital has been on the phone all morning with your insurance company. Yesterday they approved your stay here, but this morning they called the office and said that they have changed their minds. They say that you didn't go to an approved hospital and they want to move you to another hospital in Salt Lake City. Now you can choose to do this and I'm sure they will be able to help you there, but you need to know that I don't have privileges at that hospital. If you move, I can't continue on as your therapist."

Rozanne felt her stomach drop and her heart begin to pound as she listened. She had only met Dr. Beall yesterday, but inexplicably, she felt terrified to leave him. She felt horrified at the prospects of going to another hospital. The room began to spin and the objects in the tiny room faded away from view. "Who would treat me?" she asked.

"I don't know," he answered. "Probably someone on their staff."

She began to hyperventilate. "I don't get it," she wailed. "I specifically asked over and over when I was admitted if it would be all right with my insurance company. The guy up front told me that they treat patients from my insurance company here all of the time. Why won't they approve my stay?"

Dr. Beall and Marjorie exchanged looks that sent cold chills down Rozanne's back.

Dr. Beall discreetly continued, "The insurance company claims that you tried to circumvent their procedures. They said that you should have called their 1-800 number when you needed help."

"What 1-800 number?" she asked desperately. "I didn't know there is a 1-800 number!"

"That doesn't matter to them. The woman we talked to said that when you called in to make an appointment you were difficult and wouldn't work with her."

Confused, Rozanne stammered, "But Dr. Beall I told you what happened! She was pressuring me and my students were coming and I couldn't think. I called back after school. I made an appointment. I went there and saw Peter on Saturday. I tried to be good. I tried to follow the rules. What else could I do? I just don't understand this...How could it be happening? We can't afford this…We can't afford this…" Rozanne began to keen, rocking back and forth in her chair while crying silently. "Why do these things always happen to us? I don't understand. Why do these things *always* happen to *us*?"

"Rozanne, what's going on in your head, right now?" asked Dr. Beall.

Rozanne continued to rock back and forth. "I'm thinking."

"Thinking what?" he asked.

Rozanne rocked back and forth, back and forth.

She felt the pressure of tears welling up in her eyes.

She felt the hot, sticky drops as they began to drizzle down her cheeks.

She felt the room growing smaller and smaller.

She felt a thick, dark mist choke her as she struggled for air.

Just when she felt that she would slide down the deep, dark hole from which there is no return, she managed to say, "I'm thinking that I should have done it while I had the chance."

Dr. Beall and Marjorie exchanged concerned looks and Dr. Beall told Rozanne that they would be right back. They left the room and Rozanne rocked back and forth, back and forth…"I should have done it…I should have done it…We'll never be able to pay this back. It's all my fault…Oh, it's all my fault."

After a while, Dr. Beall returned and said softly, his voice ringing with amazement. "Rozanne, something has happened that I've never seen before. The hospital has agreed to keep you here, even though they know the insurance might never pay them. In all my years of practicing, I've never seen a hospital be willing to do this. They feel that your care would be too compromised. They feel that it would be devastating to you to move you, so they've agreed to keep you here and let me continue to treat you."

Rozanne stopped rocking. She took in long, deep breaths of cool air. She stared straight ahead and tried to understand what he had told her. He asked her, "What are you thinking now?"

"Don't cry," she replied.

"Why shouldn't you cry?" he asked.

She answered without emotion, "Because big girls don't cry."

"What else?"

"Pull yourself up by your bootstraps," she said, her eyes remaining fixed ahead.

"Do you really believe that?"

She nodded firmly, eyes still in place. "It's what I'm supposed to do."

"What if it's too hard?" she heard him say.

She shook her head impatiently. "That's not the issue."

"No, I think that is the issue," Dr. Beall said. "What if it is too hard for one person to do it? What if you need help?"

Rozanne thought about his questions briefly, but she couldn't process them. Discouraged, she sighed, "Nobody can help me."

"Why not?"

"Because…Because I'm supposed to get tough…" she claimed. "I'm supposed to not get so upset. I'm supposed to have more faith than this."

"I am interested in all of these things you are supposed to do," Dr. Beall said. "Do you think you could make a list of these things for me?"

Rozanne broke her fixed gaze and looked over at him. "What do you mean?"

"I want you to think of all of the things that your head is telling you that you are supposed to be thinking and doing. Then we'll go over the list and see if it makes any sense. Do you think you could do that?"

"I guess so."

"Good. I have something for you."

He leaned over and pulled a small journal out of his briefcase. It was about 8" by 5" and was covered with beautiful fruit and vines on a trellis. The artwork was done in colored pencils and Rozanne liked the way the artist had used purple to do the shading with instead of black. It made her feel peaceful just to look at it.

"I like it—a lot," she said, contentedly rubbing the journal with her hand. It felt smooth and silky and comforting to stroke the cover of the book.

He smiled. "I thought you might. It reminded me of you, somehow."

Rozanne thought that that was an interesting thing to say. Maybe other people saw her differently than she saw herself. "Dr. Beall, what's next?" she asked, still admiring her new journal.

"You just work on your list and I'll worry about that," he instructed.

"Okay," she said, pacified for the moment.

Gloria was waiting for her when she emerged from her session with Dr. Beall. "Oh, good! I was hoping you'd get through soon! It's time for lunch. Are you ready to come?"

"Just a minute, Rozanne replied. "I have to put this in my room."

"Okay," nodded Gloria. "Can I come?"

"Sure."

They walked together down the hall and Gloria chattered about what she was planning to do when she went home. She had decided to go to college. She wasn't sure what she would study, but she wanted to try it anyway. Did Rozanne think that was a good idea?

"I think you owe it to yourself to give it a try," she answered. "If you don't, you'll always wonder if you could have done it. The worse thing that could happen is you won't like it. There are tutors and programs to help students who find that it is hard for them, but who are willing to work hard to succeed. Just go to the counseling center and ask."

Gloria skipped slightly. "I was hoping you'd say that. I'm going to make some phone calls this afternoon."

"Why don't you try the community college first?" Rozanne instructed. "They're used to having older students come back to give it a try."

"That's a good idea," Gloria said. "Thanks!"

When they came out of Rozanne's room, Mark was waiting for them with the rest of the group. "Are you two ready to go?" he asked. Then, without waiting for a reply, he led the group down the hall, pushed the large metal circle that buzzed them through to the outer hall and escorted them down to the cafeteria.

As they ate, Rozanne asked Andy what he did for a living. "I'm an electronics technician."

"Really?" Rozanne said. "My husband used to do that when he was in the Air Force. How long have you been doing it?"

Andy finished the bite in his mouth before answering. "For about five years," he said at last, wiping his mouth with a napkin. "When I was living in California I worked in construction. One day a beam fell on me and hurt my back and I couldn't lift heavy loads anymore. Workman's Compensation Insurance helped me get retrained so that I could still work for a living and not have to be on disability."

""I didn't know that Workman's Comp will do that," Rozanne said.

Andy took another bite of his sandwich, chewed and swallowed it. After he had gulped half a glass of milk he continued, "That was in California. Every state is different. I don't know if they do that here in Utah."

They continued eating. Rozanne dug into a big piece of German chocolate cake. It was dry. "Too bad," she thought. "It looked so good…" Her thoughts were interrupted by Andy's voice, "My wife is coming to see me tonight."

She looked up to see Andy staring away into the distance. "Is that a good thing or a bad thing?" she asked.

"I'm not sure," he answered. "I want her to believe me when I say how much I want to change and never drink again. I want her to believe that this time is going to be different, but I don't know if she'll be able to believe me. I've let her down so many times before."

Rozanne reached over and placed her hand on the edge of his tray. "I guess that you'll just have to show her, huh?"

"Yes. It's gonna be tough, though. I just don't know how she'll be tonight. I'm scared."

"I can tell," Rozanne told him. "Just talking about it is making you shake."

Andy held up his right hand and watched it as tremors moved it without his permission. "The shaking is not all about that—although it's probably part of it. I drank for so long that I'm shaking now because I'm drying out. The doctor says it will go away in a little while, but it's annoying."

Andy made a fist with his hand and clenched it tightly before pounding the table in dismay. "My body is crying out for a drink, but my mind says, "No, not this time." I've just got to beat it or I'm going to lose my family. I've got too much at stake."

During free time, Rozanne asked a staff member for a pencil and began working on the list Dr. Beall had assigned. Closing her eyes, she allowed her mind to roam freely, listening for the inner instructions she carried with her daily. She thought the assignment would be difficult, but was surprised that the list was almost too easy to complete. The instructions were there, firmly imbedded in her mind.

Tapes In My Head

Be good.
Do your best.
If you have to look some way, why not look your best?
Keep it in the family.
Don't cry.
Don't get mad.
Don't talk back.
Listen to your mother.
Mothers take the smallest piece.
Children come first.
All children should have music lessons.
Iron your husband's shirts.
You should get up every morning and make your husband breakfast.

Never say "no" to your husband.

The mother should put the children to bed at night.

If you can't say anything nice, don't say anything at all.

Children should be seen—not heard.

We don't do THAT in OUR family.

These doctors give out too much medicine. Are you sure you (or your child) REALLY need to take all of that stuff? People didn't need it during my day and they were better off.

Pull up your bootstraps.

It's woman's work.

People hate you when you make mistakes. They won't forgive you and will talk about it amongst themselves.

Mom's way is the righteous way.

What will the neighbors say?

"That's enough," she said to herself, slamming the journal shut. "That's enough of that for today. It makes me feel like a traitor to write all of this down. It makes me feel so incredibly guilty."

Rozanne glanced at her watch and realized that it was nearly time for the afternoon Substance Abuse group. Picking up the journal and pencil, she left her room. As she walked down the hall she could hear some voices coming from inside the staff room. Someone had accidentally left the window open.

"Dr. Morrison is just about ready to send Tawny to the state," said a female voice.

"I know, I heard," replied a male voice. "She won't eat or do anything for herself."

"It's too bad," added the first voice, "but we're running out of ideas here. He's got to do something."

Rozanne slipped into the group room before the owners of the voices could look up and discover that she'd heard them. She found it empty except for Heather.

"Heather…Heather," she whispered. "Tawny's doctor is thinking about sending her to the state hospital."

"You're kidding!" Heather quietly exclaimed. "How come?"

Rozanne looked back at the doorway. They were still alone. "Because they can't get her to eat or anything. We've got to do something about it."

Heather nodded. "Let's go find Tawny," she said.

They crept back down the hall, Heather leading the way. Tawny's room was two doors down and across the hall from Rozanne's. It was dark inside. Heather threw on the light switch and rushed to Tawny's bed.

Tawny was lying in the center, curled up in her customary position. Heather sat down next to her and poked her, "Tawny…Tawny…Tawny! You've got to get up! You've got to get dressed. You've got to go down the hall and eat something. They're going to send you away…. Do you hear me? They're going to send you away!"

"Go away," Tawny mumbled.

"Tawny, I'm not going away!" Heather said. "This is too important. You've got to listen to me. Why do you want to go home so bad?"

"I want to see my son," Tawny complained. "They won't let me see him. He's just little. I need to go home, but they won't let me."

Heather sighed irritably. "Well, you're going about this all wrong! Lying around in your bathrobe, curled up in a ball is just going to get you committed to the state hospital. Is that what you want? If you go there you won't see your son for a long, long time."

"I want to go home," Tawny moaned.

Rozanne walked to the other side of the bed and knelt down by Tawny. "It's true, Tawny. I overheard them talking about it myself. If you don't get up, get dressed and eat something, they're going to send you away. Come on Tawny. You can do it. Do it for your son. He needs his mom."

Tawny stared into Rozanne's eyes before rolling away to bury her head in a pillow. She began to cry silently, her shoulders heaving up and down. When she was through, she suddenly sat up.

"That's good, Tawny!" Heather said, "That's real good. It's a beginning. Now we're going to go down to group. You get dressed and come down when you're ready. Then you walk in the room and you sit up and you look at Carol right in the eye. You listen to the conversation. You even say a few things. You got it?"

"Yes."

Heather patted her on the shoulder. "Good. We'll see you down there in a minute. Do it, Tawny. Do it for your son."

Rozanne and Heather arrived at the group room to discover that the Substance Abuse meeting was already in session. "Where were you two?" said Carol.

Heather answered for them. "I was showing Rozanne some drawings my kids did for me and we lost track of time. Sorry."

"That's okay," replied Carol." Come on in and join us."

When they were settled, Carol looked around the room and said, "Now, where were we? Oh, I remember—I was talking to you about coping skills. We all need to learn better ways to deal with anxiety and stress. This is particularly important for individuals in your situation. When you become adept at using these techniques, you don't have to feel nervous and upset when something bad happens to you. You can learn to relax, instead of overreact. You can learn to let go of the tension you feel in productive ways. Any questions?"

Carol could see that they weren't going to respond, so she continued, "The first thing you have to do when using these techniques is make a list of things that stress you out. Next, you make a list of things that you can say to yourself to get through these stressful events. Are you with me?" she said to them.

When no one indicated otherwise, Carol walked over to the whiteboard and picked up a red marker. "Let's start by making list of negative things you say to yourself when you are facing hard times," Carol told them. "Any ideas?"

Silence.

Carol encouraged, "Come on. I'll bet someone here has something that can get us going."

"I can't do it," said Gloria, frustrated.

"Good! That's the idea, Gloria!"

Gloria turned red and wrung her hands together. "Why are you making fun of me?"

"I'm not making fun of you, Gloria," Carol quickly said. "Why do you think I am?"

Gloria looked confused. "Because you said it's a good thing that I can't do it."

Colby snickered.

Carol ignored him. "No, Gloria. That's not what I said. When you said that you couldn't do it, I thought you were giving us an example. As it turns out, you were giving us a perfect example. The "I can't do it" statement you made is one of those statements that aren't helpful. You can do it, Gloria, but you tell yourself that you can't. What happens when you say that?"

Gloria looked at the other patients. They were all staring at her. She squirmed and answered, "I feel stupid."

Carol wrote, "I feel stupid" on the board under "I can't do it" before turning to Gloria. "What else?" she encouraged.

"I get sort of…a…well…nervous," Gloria answered.

"Good…go on," Carol said, taking down Gloria's reply.

Gloria started to understand what Carol was trying to show them. She thought a minute longer before saying triumphantly, "I start to feel depressed!"

Carol grinned at her. "Exactly! Gloria, you're making my point beautifully. Thanks for your help. The statement, "I can't do it" increases your stress reactions. If you can learn to substitute more helpful statements like, 'This may be tough, but I've done tough things before' or, 'It's easier once you get started' or, 'I can do this,' you'll find that that your body and mind starts to relax and you feel that you can cope with the situation. Do you understand now?"

"Oh, I get it!" Gloria exclaimed. "If I say, 'I can't do it,' then my body reacts and I really can't do it!"

Carol nodded at Gloria happily before turning to Colby and asking, "Colby, how could this information be of use to you?"

Colby sneered. "I don't have a clue. I don't want to get a clue either."

Carol sighed and asked Andy the same question. Andy thought briefly before replying, "If I could learn to stop saying those kind of things to myself, I could get myself through situations where I normally would over-react…Like the times I want to go on a bender…or the times I get mad and blow up at my kids because they're fighting over something stupid."

"That's right," Carol said. "You've got it."

The discussion was interrupted by the sound of Macie gasping for air. "Look who's coming!" she burst out. "I can't believe it. I can't believe it…"

They turned to look in the direction Macie was pointing. To their amazement they saw Tawny, fully dressed with her hair combed, walking down the hall towards them. She was slightly bent over, as if she didn't want to be noticed, but she was walking with more confidence than they'd ever seen. Tawny entered the room and looked over at Rozanne and Heather. Heather gave her a wink and Rozanne smiled at her. Then Tawny simply said, "Sorry I'm late."

Carol stared at her, dumbfounded. After she collected herself, she said to Tawny, "It's okay, really…Why don't you sit down?"

Heather patted the couch next to her and said, "Come on over by me, Tawny."

Macie announced, "Well, I'll be sniggered. What got into her?" Rozanne reached over and gave Macie a little kick with a look that said, "You better stop it right now!" Macie gulped and looked down at her hands and then began picking fuzz off of the navy-blue sweats she was wearing.

Carol hesitated just a second before beginning again, "…It's like we were saying before you came in, Tawny, if you can just learn to replace negative self-talk with positive self-talk, you can get yourself through situations that normally cause you to drink, do drugs, or get depressed. Now, I would like to go on and have us make a list of these positive stress-coping thoughts. Are you ready?"

Heather answered for the rest of them. "Carol, why don't you go ahead?"

Carol took her eyes away from Tawny. Nodding at Heather she answered, "Okay, I will. To understand how this works you've got to know about the four steps we all go through when we respond to something emotionally."

Carol picked up the eraser and wiped away the list she had been making. As she continued lecturing, she wrote down pertinent facts on the board to emphasize their importance. Once she had completed the oration the board looked like this:

1. Something happens—like your boss gets mad at you or your forget to get something really important at the store, etc.
2. Your body reacts—You start to sweat, you shake, you feel a tight, icky feeling in your stomach, you feel dizzy.
3. You do something—like trying to apologize or try to get away from the situation as quickly as you can. You may get a drink. You may get a fix. You may isolate yourself.
4. You think something—You say negative things like "I can't stand it…It's hopeless…I'm at my limit…I'm losing it…" to yourself. Then you start to feel the emotions that follow those statements. Examples of these emotions are hopelessness, fear, and anger…

Carol stood back and admired her work. Turning slightly, she looked back toward the patients and asked, "Do any of you have examples you can give about how you react in situations that stress you out?"

"I curl up in a ball and refuse to talk," Tawny said, hesitantly.

Everyone was stunned, most of all Carol.

Then Tawny started to giggle. It just bubbled up like a mountain spring and pretty soon, Heather and Rozanne were laughing, too. As she laughed, Tawny covered her mouth as if she was trying to hide the delight inside, but her eyes twinkled and betrayed her. Carol was disconcerted by this sudden turn of events and flashed indignant looks at Heather and Rozanne, but they just kept laughing. After all, they were the only ones who knew what was so funny.

At dinner that night, Rozanne finally got a good look at Laura. She had shoulder length, medium-brown hair and an olive complexion. She was eating her meal with a man about her same age, which Rozanne guessed to be in the mid-twenties. The man, who Rozanne supposed was Laura's husband, was talking with animation to her, but Laura was staring out the window as if she didn't realize he was there. He was trying to ignore this lack of interest on her part and seemed to be overcompensating for her apathy. When Laura finished her food, she stood and walked back down the hall to the ward. Her husband hurriedly emptied the trays and then ran down the hall to catch her.

Rozanne watched all of this with deep curiosity. What was going on with her, anyway? Why didn't she have to live by the same rules as everybody else? They couldn't leave the cafeteria until everyone was ready to go. They had to be with a staff member whenever they were off of the ward. Laura seemed to go and do whatever she pleased. It also puzzled Rozanne that no one else seemed to notice or pay attention to the "Laura" mystery. It was almost like Laura didn't exist.

"Rozanne, can you hurry and finish eating? You have some visitors back on the wing."

Rozanne looked up to see someone she didn't recognize. It was a woman about fifty-five with short, dyed, red hair. She had a pleasant look on her face.

"Who are you?" Rozanne wondered out loud.

"Oh, sorry," the woman said. "I thought you knew. I'm Kris Stanworth. I'm on the evening shift tonight. I'll be here with you until about noon tomorrow. Are you ready to go?"

"Hi, honey," Gary said as he kissed her. "I ran into Bishop Finlinson on the way in. That was good timing, wasn't it?"

"It sure was," answered the bishop as he reached out to shake Rozanne's hand. "I was starting to feel lost when Gary stumbled across me. This place is a maze. How are you doing? I've been so worried about you. Toni told me that the kids at school are lost without you."

"Toni?" asked Gary.

"That's Sister Larson's first name, Gary," informed Rozanne.

"Oh," he murmured.

"This is really tough, Bishop," Rozanne said. "I never thought I'd end up in a place like this. It's not so bad, though, and I think I really need to be here. I feel safe for the first time in quite a while."

Bishop Finlinson nodded as he visually scanned the area. "I'm surprised myself at how nice this place is. It's not what I expected at all." Looking back at her he added, "Should we get to the real reason I came? Is there somewhere private we can go?"

"I don't know. I'll ask," replied Rozanne.

She went over to the staff window and asked Kris about their needs. Kris brought out a key and let them into the same room Rozanne that had her counseling sessions with Dr. Beall.

Rozanne and Gary took two chairs that were next to each other and Gary reached out and took her hand in his. The bishop sat across from

Rozanne. He looked back and forth at their faces before saying, "I'm concerned about your family. Will you let us bring in meals while you are in the hospital?"

"All right," Rozanne said. "It will make things easier for Gary. But did he tell you that I don't want anybody to know?"

"Yes, he told me. Lisa is going to have all of the meals delivered to our home and then she'll take them to your house. Is that all right?"

"Lisa? Oh, that's right. Your wife is the Compassionate Service Leader," Rozanne said, relieved.

"Lisa will also call you as soon as you get home so we can decide what you need then, okay?" said the bishop.

"Okay."

"What about your Visiting Teachers?" he asked. "Don't you want them to know?"

"No!" she said. "If I ever decide to tell them, I want it to be my decision. I don't want to take the chance that they'll gossip."

"I don't know that I agree, but I'll honor your wishes, Rozanne. Now what about the bill for the hospital. Do you have insurance?"

"We do," she sighed, "but they're refusing to pay the bill. The hospital has agreed to let me stay anyway. I'm not sure what will happen now."

"You know that we can help you with fast offerings, if you need us to," he informed.

Gary and Rozanne looked at each other. "No, I didn't know that," she replied carefully. She didn't like the idea of the ward having to bail them out. It felt humiliating.

Bishop Finlinson leaned forward in his chair and instructed, "You need this care and we will support you in making sure that you receive it. You and Gary try to do your best to take care of things and then, if you need some help, I want you to promise me that you'll ask."

"I promise," she said, although she didn't really mean it.

He studied her thoughtfully. "Are you ready for a blessing now?"

"More than you'll ever know."

At the conclusion of her blessing, Rozanne went to find Gloria. She was waiting impatiently for Rozanne in the day room. "Gloria, my Bishop is here. Do you still want a blessing?"

Gloria jumped up and rushed towards her. "Oh, yes. I was hoping you hadn't forgotten. Can we go right now?"

"Of course."

"Would you stay with me while I have it?" Gloria pleaded.

Rozanne smiled, "If you'd like me to."

After Rozanne introduced Gloria to Bishop Finlinson, he asked Gloria to tell him a little about herself. She told him about her mission to Colorado. She completed her mission in good standing, but she began struggling with depression after she returned home. She had feelings of not being smart enough…not being worthy enough…and she couldn't seem to shake them off. She told Bishop Finlinson about her problems and about the mistakes she'd made. She also told him about the progress she'd made since coming to the hospital and that she'd been reading the Book of Mormon ever since Rozanne gave her a copy the night before.

Bishop Finlinson listened carefully and then said, "Gloria, you must promise me that after you're released from the hospital you'll make every effort to find your own bishop and speak with him. Let him help you. He's the Lord's representative for you. The Lord has given him the keys and authority to help you find the answers you need. He'll help guide you through the repentance process. He'll help you as you walk the path back to full activity. Don't underestimate his ability to love you in spite of your problems. Will you promise me to do this?"

Gloria studied her hands momentarily before meeting his gaze. "Yes," she resolved.

Bishop Finlinson nodded his endorsement of her reply. "Good. Don't deny yourself the source of true happiness. You'll find it through following the teachings of the Savior, Jesus Christ. Now, are you ready for a blessing?" Turning his gaze to Gary he continued, "Brother Paxman, would you anoint and I'll bless, if that's all right with you, Gloria."

At the conclusion of the blessing Gloria looked up, her eyes shining. "Oh, thank you. That's the first time I've felt the spirit in such a long time. I know what I need to do now. I need to see my bishop and I need to go home and make peace with my parents. I believe that I can make it if I can remember what I used to try to teach other people. Jesus Christ lived and died for me. I've got to remember that…I'd forgotten that he loves even me."

When the men had left to return home, Gloria and Rozanne went into the group room to talk. They were sitting, side by side, on the long couch discussing the blessings they had been given when Heather entered the room. She sat down at the table behind the couch and began coloring the picture she had been working on for two days. As Gloria and Rozanne continued their conversation Heather began to eavesdrop. "Rozanne," Gloria inquired, "have you ever truly given up on life?"

Rozanne considered her question. She tried to remember how she felt when she was suicidal. It was so dark in that closet—so dark…She could still feel the heaviness of the coats hanging in front of her face. She could still smell the stale air of the confined space. She tried to remember. "No," she said at last. "I guess not. Even when I've thought it was totally hopeless there was always a part of me that told me I needed to keep going—that there is a reason I'm here and that I've got to keep trying, no matter how hard it feels at the moment. I think if I had truly given up, I would have driven my van off of the road that day or swallowed something when I got home. But that part of me, the part that keeps going wouldn't let me. "It" stopped me from hurting myself. "It" got me home. "It" made me realize I needed to come here. "It" tells me to work hard at getting better."

Gloria chewed on her thumbnail as she examined Rozanne's profile. "What is 'it'?" Rozanne bit her lip and thought. Deliberately she replied, "I believe that "it" is my spirit. My spirit remembers being with Heavenly Father before we came to earth. My spirit remembers why I'm here and wants more than anything to go home. It's my body that wants to give up. It's my body that wants to listen to Satan and destroy itself. But so far, my spirit has won the battle. My spirit remembers Jesus Christ and knows that he loves me and wants to help me. My spirit wants me to repent and change."

Gloria bowed her head and asked, "How do you know that?"

Rozanne turned to her and answered, "Remember who it was that testified to the people on your mission that what they were hearing was true?"

Gloria brightened as she remembered the answer. "Oh, yes! I know that! It's the Holy Ghost!"

"That's right," Rozanne returned. "The Holy Ghost tells us when we are right or wrong. If we don't ignore him, we can get better and better at hearing what he is saying. He testifies to us of Christ and Heavenly Father. He teaches us. My problem has been that, somehow, I've let myself get so lost in the cares of my life that I've forgotten how to listen to my spirit and to the Holy Ghost. I've got to find my way back and I've got to have help because my body is in such a mess. Depression does that to you. You just get so lost…"

Heather joined them on the couch. "How do you know that?" she quizzed. "I mean, how do you know that you were with God before? What do you mean about wanting to go home? Do you want to kill yourself?"

"No, that's not what I mean at all," Rozanne answered. "My spirit remembers being at home. I can't remember it with my mind, but I think that somehow, that part of me we call our spirit can remember. Sometimes I get so homesick for Heavenly Father. But if I kill myself, I won't be able to go home. Instead it will be just the opposite. I think I may be lost forever…

Rozanne stopped, sighed, and ran her fingers through her hair. "So I've got to get the strength to stop thinking about it. The only way I can really go home and be with Heavenly Father again is if I can find a way to not only endure this life, but to embrace it with full force and to love and serve everyone I can."

Rozanne looked over at Gloria and Heather. They were studying her intently. She looked away and continued, "But right now I'm sick. I'm sick emotionally and I've got to get better before I can do the things I need and want to do. This sickness is sort of like cancer. It can kill. It tried to kill me once and it'll probably try again, but just like cancer there are ways to beat it and I'm going to learn what to do."

Gloria and Heather nodded in agreement. They all sat in silence, considering this idea. Then Rozanne slowly said, "I think that in some ways it's much worse than cancer. It's so real and so devastating, but people are afraid of it. No one wants to talk about it. No one wants to admit that they are seriously depressed, so they try to suffer through it alone. It's hard to admit that you need help…"

Rozanne looked over at Heather. She had her head buried in her legs. Rozanne sighed, "And a lot of people, frankly, are quite judgmental. I've heard people in different wards I've lived in gossip about this sister or that sister who was depressed. They pass harsh judgement of these individuals. Some people think that all depressed people need to do to get better is to get up and start smiling…count their blessings and they'll feel fine. I don't think…no, I know…it's not always that simple. I think that's why so many people end up losing the battle in the end. They're too ashamed to ask for help. I know I was. I'm glad that I'm finally on the road to recovery, even though I'm sure it's going to be a long and rocky road that leads up a very steep hill."

Day 3

▼

"Macie! Macie! Where are you? You come out of wherever you hiding! You're just going to make trouble for yourself, Macie"

Kris stood in the hall for a moment and thought, "Where in the world could she be? I just went to the bathroom for a minute and when I came out she was gone. If I don't find her soon we're going to have to do something drastic with her. Now, let's see…I checked the day room and the group room. I looked in her room and her bathroom. I looked out on the smoking terrace.…"

CRASH! A loud noise came from Macie's room that sounded like someone was trying to push down the wall. Kris bolted back down the hall and into Macie's room to discover Macie sprawled on the bathroom floor with the towel bar in her right hand. Her left hand was on her forehead and she was bellowing like a cow past milking time.

"Kris, what's going on?" yelled Mark, following her down the hall.

"Oh, it's just Macie," Kris said. "She slipped away from me when I went to powder my nose and I've been looking for her. Macie, where in heaven's name were you hiding?"

Macie stuck her tongue out at them. "Don't you wish you knew? Ha! You'll never get it out of me."

Mark reached down to pull Macie off of the floor while instructing, "Now, Macie let's get you back down to the day room and we can decide what we're going to do about this. What were you doing with the towel bar anyway?"

"I was going to make a club to beat you with!"

"Ha, ha," Mark replied. "Macie, you can't go around saying things like that. We'll have to put that in your chart."

"Can't you take a joke?" Macie muttered. "I was only kidding."

Kris rolled her eyes at Mark. "So you were kidding. Will you get up and come with us now?" she demanded.

Macie rolled over and slowly got on her knees. She rocked back and forth for a few moments before Kris took her arm and assisted her to her feet. Then Mark and Kris each took an arm and they helped Macie stumble back down to the day room and seated her at the table.

Kris faced Macie, deposited her hands on her hips and demanded, "Are you ready to tell us what was going on back there?"

"No!" Macie snarled.

Kris sighed and looked at Mark across the top of Macie's head. He shook his head in return. Kris continued the interrogation, "You realize, of course, that we're going to have to call your doctor about what you did? Why don't you make things easier and tell us what you were thinking about when you ran away from me? Why were you hiding? Where were you hiding?"

Macie folded her arms defiantly. "You two think you know everything…Ha! I guess I showed you, didn't I? Well, sorry to disappoint you…I'll tell my doctor in person what I was doing…. And that is that!"

Mark got down on one knee and looked Macie in the eyes. Macie stared back at Mark for sometime before averting her eyes. Mark sighed and asked, "Macie, if we let you go to group this morning, will you promise to be good? Will you promise to stay in line of sight of staff at all times?"

"All right, all right," she relented. "Just let me go to group, will ya?"

Macie got up and started walking towards the door. She stopped, looked back at Mark and Kris, who were still sitting at the round table and in a tone that mimicked a young child mocked, "Mother, may I go to group now?"

"Yes, Macie," they replied in unison.

Rhaun was writing a series of statements on the white board when Macie entered the room. He continued writing as he remarked, "Hi, Macie. Find a place and sit down."

Macie looked around the room. Rozanne already took up her favorite corner of the big leather couch. Gloria was on the other end and Tawny was sitting right in the middle of the short leather couch with Andy on her left. Colby, Heather and Lizbeth were coloring at the table. But there was someone new. He looked like he was a Native American and he was sitting in the big armchair she sometimes liked to take.

"Hey, Rhaun. Who's the new guy?" she demanded.

Rhaun stopped writing and turned to look at her. "Macie, if you'd been on time you'd already know. This is Howard. He checked in during the night."

She squinted at Howard. "Howard, huh? Hey, Howard. What ya in for?"

Howard looked around as if he didn't know what to say. Andy caught his eye and smiled encouragingly at him. Finally, he answered Macie, "I guess I'm here because I'm a drunk."

"Substance abuse," corrected Andy.

"Substance abuse," Howard repeated.

Macie sauntered over to the long couch and plunked down in middle, sprawling her arms and legs out enough to make Rozanne and Gloria feel quite uncomfortable before she continued her interrogation of Howard, "You an Indian or something?"

"I'm a Navajo," replied Howard.

"Navajo…oh yeah," sniffed Macie. "I know that. That's a tribe, right?"

"Yes, that's a tribe," Howard answered evenly.

Macie absentmindedly scratched her scalp before looking at her finger to see if there was any evidence of dandruff on it. "Where ya from?" she asked.

Howard looked around for help, but instead saw a room full of people staring inquisitively at him. "New Mexico, originally," he informed her. "About 30 miles northeast of Farmington."

Macie yawned. "I don't know where that is, but it doesn't matter."

Rhaun had listened to enough. "Macie, we are talking about stopping irrational ideas. Do you know what that means?"

Macie tapped her foot impatiently on the floor, bouncing the other occupants of the couch with her. "Nope," she said in a manner that indicated the idea totally bored her.

Rhaun studied Macie briefly before shaking his head in irritation. "Macie, almost every minute of your whole life you are talking to yourself in your head. If you're talking to yourself in terms that are reasonable, then you're okay. But the problem with some—a lot—of people that have depression and abuse problems is that they talk to themselves in irrational ways."

"What do you mean by irrational?" Macie said as she tried to sneak a peak at Rozanne's journal. Rozanne pulled it closer to stop the prying eyes from seeing what she was writing.

"Irrational—out of touch with reality…untrue…It's self-talk that makes the situation you are dealing with seem…oh, sort of impossible to deal with," Rhaun answered.

Macie shrugged her shoulders as she reluctantly pulled herself back to her original position. "Oh, yeah. I probably got that."

"Yes, Macie, I believe you probably do," Rhaun concluded. "What we're doing right now is making a list of some statements that the group has come up with that are irrational."

Macie looked at the board. It read:

- I better not say anything that upsets anyone.
- Why do terrible things always happen to me?
- I'm not a good person.
- People always ignore me.
- I'm ugly.
- I can't fail or everyone will hate me.
- It's impossible to overcome my past mistakes.
- I want everyone to like me.
- People who do wrong things don't deserve to be loved.
- When I make a mistake, I ruin the lives of the people I love.
- Life is unfair.

Rhaun looked over at Rozanne and asked, "Rozanne, can you think of anything else?"

Rozanne looked blankly at Rhaun for a moment before he continued, trying to help jog her thought process. "We've been talking about something in group that you experience that can be easily traced to these types of statements. Think a minute," he coaxed, "take your time…"

"Do you mean about feeling guilty all of the time?" she smiled.

"Bingo! No one does things worth feeling guilty about all of the time. There have to be some redeeming moments. I want you to think of an irrational self-talk statement you say to yourself. Try to pick one that probably isn't true, even though it makes you feel guilty anyway. Can you do it?"

"I'll try."

"Good. You sit there and think about it for a while and when you're ready you tell us what it is."

"Rhaun, I think I have something," she replied immediately.

"What is it?" he asked.

"If your child doesn't do well in school it means you're stupid and a failure and you need to feel guilty for letting everybody down."

Rhaun's eyes flew open. "Where did that come from? Are you really carrying that kind of thing around in your head?"

"I guess so..."

Rhaun shook his head in dismay. "You know what you need to do? Write down some of those statements in your journal. Then you can look at them rationally and see if they make sense."

"That's funny...that's what Dr. Beall told me to do."

"Well, you know what they say about great minds, don't you?" Rhaun laughed.

"Ha, ha, Rhaun...Do you really think you have a great mind?" Colby snorted.

"How about you Colby?" Rhaun shot back. "What irrational self-talk is going on in that head of yours?"

"My head?" Colby sneered. "You'll never know. My head is a closed book."

Lizbeth giggled, "Colby, I don't think that book has ever been opened before."

Gloria added, "That's right, Colby. That book has never even left the library!"

Colby pulled a face at Lizbeth before returning to work on his picture as if nothing happened.

Andy jumped in, "Rhaun, I think I may have something for you. I was just thinking...When I come home and the kids are fussing, like kids do, and my wife hasn't made dinner, and my boss has been yammering at me and so on, I think that I use this crazy self-talk to convince myself that it's okay to drink.

"That's reasonable," Rhaun agreed. "Do you want to give us some examples of what you tell yourself?"

"How about this," Andy started. "I can't take it. Why can't Sylvia keep things in control? My boss hates me and there's nothing I can do about it…Maybe he'll fire me because he was yelling at me…I can't talk to him about it…it's impossible…I'd like to get another job, but I just can't do it because nothing ever goes right for me…I need a drink…I can't help the way I feel…Why can't people be better to me so I can deal with things? It's all her fault…If she'd just keep the house cleaner…If she'd take better care of the kids…I need a drink. I'll feel better. Just one drink won't matter…"

"That's quite a list, Andy," remarked Heather.

"I know." he replied. "I've never realized before that this could be part of my problem."

Rozanne jumped in. "I know what you mean, Andy. I've always believed that thoughts were something you ride, like a surfer on a big wave. Sometimes the surf is good and sometimes, well, it throws you off and you drown."

Rhaun smiled at Rozanne. "It's an amazing concept that you can do something about the surf, isn't it?"

"When will we learn how?" she asked.

"Is tomorrow soon enough?" Rhaun laughed.

"Good," Rozanne said firmly as she closed her journal and looked up at him. "That's very good."

Dr. Beall was waiting for Rozanne in the hall when the group session had ended. "I timed it just right. Are you ready to talk to me?"

"Sure," she replied easily. She followed Dr. Beall down the hall and into the room where they'd been meeting each day. When they were settled she asked, "What's on the agenda this morning?"

"I thought we'd work on clearing up some of your traumatic experiences," he told her.

"My traumatic experiences?"

"Your traumatic experiences," he repeated. "Let me explain…People who get depressed usually have had some traumatic experiences that haunt them. When we are putting someone like you back together, we need to address these things."

Rozanne furrowed her eyebrows, "Put me back together? What do you mean by that?"

Dr. Beall answered, "We can't just skip over your past and expect you to become well again. We have to start at the beginning and rebuild your life. We need to resolve issues that have been lingering like unseen ghosts in your mind."

Rozanne thought that made sense. She certainly had a few ghosts she wanted to exorcise. She squinted her eyes and quizzed, "Dr. Beall, what do you think has happened to me?"

"I think you've had what physicians used to call a nervous breakdown," he replied. "A lot of doctors don't like that term anymore, but I think it fits many people very well. After all, that's what happened. Your nervous system got strained to the point where it couldn't go on and then it shut down. I see it all of the time—especially in women."

"I've heard that before," she remarked. "Why do you think it happens so often to women?"

"Oh, don't get me wrong," Dr. Beall asserted, "it happens to men, too—even prominent community members."

"Really?"

"Sure," he replied, "they're people too, you know. When someone has a nervous breakdown they've usually tried to take on too much and their situation has buried them in stress. Their body simply says, "That's enough! If you aren't going to take care of me willingly, I'm going to force you to pay attention!" Nervous breakdowns are exactly what they sound like; the nervous system shuts down and you can't cope with life anymore."

"Do you really see it a lot?" she demanded, unwilling to accept what he was telling her.

Dr. Beall pulled a face. "More than I'd like to, that's for sure," he remarked. "I'd say it happens to women so often because life demands so much of them. They have the home, the kids, their husbands, work, the community, and their church callings—and so on and so on...A lot of women—especially Latter-day Saint women—try too hard to meet everyone's expectations of them. They want to be perfect. They get discouraged. They don't want to admit to anyone that they are doing too much, even to themselves. They have this unrealistic picture of the perfect LDS woman. She bakes bread. She sews. She does crafts. She has perfect children and lives in a completely clean home. She has time to read her scriptures, tole paints all of the doors in her home, jog five miles a day and bake Swedish Christmas bread for the neighborhood. She has three callings and baby-sits the children of the ladies she visit teaches once a month so they can go to the temple. She does genealogy. She gardens and her yard looks like it should be in a magazine layout. On top of all of that, she is a successful career woman. If she can't do all of this at one time—it means she is a failure. Add this to the hormonal problems many women experience and you have a formula for trouble."

"I can certainly understand that," Rozanne agreed. "It sounds just like me. So what do we do now?"

Dr. Beall leaned back in his chair and contemplated her question. "My job is to help you find answers and give you tools. Part of what you need to do is to decide what things are the most important to you. Then you have to discover that maybe you can do most of what you'd like to do—but just not all at the same time! I'd like you to work on a mission statement for yourself."

"What's that?"

"A mission statement is a brief statement in which you outline what is most important to you and what your ultimate goals are. It helps clear up the decision making process if you've predetermined what you value the most."

"Do you have a mission statement, Dr. Beall?"

"Yes," he replied, "but my mission statement probably is much different than yours will be. You have to determine for yourself what you value. It is very helpful.

But getting back to the trauma issues, Rozanne. I'm sure that there are some things in your life that have been troubling you…things that you just can't seem to get rid of, no matter how hard you've tried." Dr. Beall leaned in towards her. "Am I right?"

"Well, yes, you are," she said, rubbing her forehead. "But there are some things that I don't want to talk about. It makes me feel too upset. There is at least one thing that I've never told anyone about before—even Gary."

Dr. Beall sat back in his chair and smiled. "That's the beauty of the treatment I'm going to offer you. I have studied a method of treating trauma that doesn't require the patient to describe to the therapist out loud what has happened to them. All you have to do is get the picture in your mind of what happened to you and then I teach you a simple motion that processes the information. It sort of acts like an eraser. You still know what happened to you—you haven't forgotten it at all—but this treatment allows your mind to process it and the "picture" of the event fades away and you don't feel traumatized by it anymore. Do you think you could do that?"

"It's really that simple?"

"It really is," he assured. "I see patients nearly every day that have had terrible things happen to them…sexual abuse…witnessing murders…car accidents…and more. The trauma of their experiences has caused them untold amounts of pain. I teach them this method of processing memories and with my help, they learn to "erase" the picture of the event. It works so well that sometimes I even do it to myself after a session where a patient has described horrible things to me and I feel upset. I'll go in my room and do it and then I can go on and feel better."

"Okay," she agreed. "Can we get started?"

He held up his hand. "There's just one more thing we have to do before we start. It's something you have to promise me. You have to promised that you'll never teach this to someone else."

"Why?"

He explained, "Because if this motion, which is so simple, is not used correctly it can make the patient worse. You're not a therapist. A therapist who is trained in the technique needs to teach the patient how to use it correctly. Once you learn how to use it, however, you'll find it a very helpful tool. So, do you promise not to show anybody else?"

"Okay," Rozanne agreed. "I'll have trust you on that. I promise."

"Good," he smiled. "Now get a picture in your head of something that has always bothered you."

"All right. I have something." Rozanne said. She knew just where she wanted to start.

"Would you like to share anything about the incident?" asked Dr. Beall.

"I was sexually abused as a little girl. The memory of it has bothered me for years. The funny thing about it is that I had totally forgotten about what happened until I was married about a year. Then, out of the blue, I remembered. I felt sick and upset. I couldn't believe I'd forgotten something like that. I couldn't tell Gary what had happened. I could only tell him that something happened and who did it."

Dr. Beall lamented. "That's really not that uncommon. You finally remembered it at a time you felt safe. Don't worry. You don't have to tell me any details."

"Good," she said. "Other people have tried to get me to talk about it, but I didn't want to. I just can't make myself talk about it."

"I understand. Now, I want you to get the picture of what happened to you in your head. Remember the room. Remember the furniture. Remember the wallpaper, if there was any. Remember how you felt. Can you picture it?"

Rozanne felt the room changing. Yes, she remembered that room, all too well. She nodded to indicate she was following his directions.

"Now look at me and I'll show you what to do," he instructed.

After Dr. Beall had shown her what to do, she was amazed. "Wow," she exclaimed. "It's just like someone took a big eraser and wiped out the middle of the picture! I can still see the edges but the center, the part that I couldn't stand to see, is gone!"

"It's astonishing, isn't it?" he agreed. "Do you want to try another one?"

"Yes! Could I work on something someone said to me when I was in high school that has haunted me for years?"

She could just see him sitting behind that big desk like he was a king, wearing his plaid jacket and sporting that old-fashioned butch haircut. He was Dr. (and oh, let's not forget the Dr.) J. Wade Degenisis. He'd recently got that Ph.D. and it was very, very important to him.

"Well, young lady," he said as he tapped his fingers together, irritated. "What makes you think you can go to college early?"

"Come on, Dr. Degenisis. I've finished all of my classes I need for graduation. There aren't any left to take. What will I do next year? I took the ACT test and got the score mandatory for early admission. I have a scholarship. All I need now is a letter from someone here at the high school to get me in."

He rocked back in his big, brown leather chair and glared at her. "Rozanne, I want you to stay and complete your senior year." He stopped talking and leaned forward, as if he was going to let her in on a secret. "In fact," he said. "I'll promise you this; if you'll stay, I'll make you Valedictorian even if you get straight F's all next year."

Rozanne was shocked. How could he promise her something like that? "It's not right," she thought to herself. "It's just not right! No one should be Valedictorian unless they earn it honestly. It wouldn't mean anything, otherwise, and it certainly wouldn't be fair to the other students."

It was at that moment—that exact moment—that she knew that she had to get out of there, no matter what it took. She replied, "No way."

He tapped his pencil on the desk and scowled at her. "You know what your problem is?" he demanded. "You're socially maladjusted."

Socially maladjusted…socially maladjusted…those two words hung over her head like the Sword of Damocles, ready to strike anytime she felt uneasy in a social situation. It had been over twenty years since she'd heard that phrase, but she used it like a club to beat herself with. If she had a disagreement with anyone for any reason at all, she'd cry to her husband, "He was right! I'm just socially maladjusted."

"Get the picture in your head," reminded Dr. Beall

Oh yes. Rozanne could see Dr. Degenisis clearly. "Okay…I see him there in his plaid jacket."

"All right, Rozanne…let's do the technique…"

"Is it gone?" she heard Dr. Beall say.

"No," she sighed, surprised. "I can still hear it."

Dr. Beall nodded. "Then let's go out of the room. What do you see before you go into the room?"

"His secretary," she said, pulling a sour face. "Oh, she was so icky to me. Even after the school board promised me that I could have my diploma, she tried to tell me I was a high school dropout."

"That ought to work," Dr. Beall remarked. "Picture her and we'll try it again."

"Is it gone?" he asked.

Rozanne shook her head, frustrated. "Nope. How come this one is so hard?"

Dr. Beall thought a minute. "Sometimes, when something is particularly stuck in there, we have to substitute a better idea for the one that is bothering you. How about we try that?"

"Okay," she answered, "but what?"

"Can you think of something that proves that what he said to you wasn't true?" he asked.

"...No..."

"Come on, Rozanne...Think...How about your life as a teacher—didn't you do well before this year?"

Rozanne remembered and smiled. "Actually I did very well. In fact, my last principal told me that I got the highest score on the teacher evaluation that anyone on the faculty ever received."

Dr. Beall nodded. "How about the kids? Did you get along with them?"

"Oh, yes!" she said. "I loved my students so much and they loved me. It used to be wonderful teaching!"

"All right then," he said. "How about this? We'll try the technique and I want you to repeat over and over to yourself in your mind, "My life as a teacher proves that that statement is untrue." Does that sound all right?"

"I think so..."

When they were through, Dr. Beall asked her how she felt.

"I don't understand how it works," she told him. "I can't hear what he said to me ringing in my head anymore. I can conjure it up again...if I really try...but whenever I do, the statement, "My life as a teacher proves that that statement is untrue," pops right into my head. Somehow I feel better. Thanks."

Dr. Beall smiled. "I think that's enough for this morning. Now what I'd like you to do is to think of a few more incidents that we could work on resolving. We can only do a few at a time. When you work on some of the things that have been bothering you, they tend to all fall apart—like a house of cards."

Lunch was Salisbury Steak with mashed potatoes. "Yuck," Rozanne thought. "The food's starting to get to me. It's typical hospital food." She picked up her tray and went to join the group at the table. As she walked, she noticed that Laura's husband was eating with her again. Laura still hadn't said two words to Rozanne, although they had been in their room alone on several occasions. Laura would either sit on her bed and look out of the window, or sit at the only desk in the room and scribble madly into her journal.

When Rozanne started to sit down, Lizbeth called, "No, Rozanne—over here by me!" After Rozanne was seated, Lizbeth started bubbling over with excitement. It seemed that her mother and boyfriend were going to bring her children to the hospital that night to visit.

"I can't wait! I made Connie's costume months ago. She's going to be a mermaid and the boys are going to be Salt and Pepper Shakers!"

"Salt and Pepper? How did you do that?"

"Oh, it was easy!" Lizbeth said, "I got them white and black sweat suits. Then I made them foam hats and covered the hats with foil and painted circle on the tops to look like the holes in a shaker. The hats make all of the difference! Cute, huh? Then I made signs to pin on the boys that say Salt and Pepper. Jason is the Salt and Jody is the Pepper. I'm so glad that mom agreed to bring them by after they do their trick or treating. It's hard enough being in here on Halloween. Is your husband going to bring in your kids?"

"No," Rozanne answered. "It's too far."

"Sorry about that..."

"Don't worry about it," Rozanne assured her. "It's not your fault."

Andy decided to change the subject. "Rozanne, I've been thinking about something. Didn't you have your trouble because of what happened to you at school?"

Rozanne looked at him. "Yes...So?"

"I've been thinking," began Andy. "Did you ever consider that maybe, just maybe, you have a Workman's Compensation case? If you do, maybe they would pay your bills. They might even be willing to re-train you if they think you can't continue on as a teacher. I don't know what the laws in Utah are, but you ought to check into it."

Rozanne let this idea take root in her mind before replying. She'd never considered this possibility before. "I never thought of it that way," she replied. "I have a card they gave me at work that tells me what to do to file a claim. Maybe I'll call them after lunch."

"Good," Andy nodded. "It's worth a try."

The group continued their conversation as they worked their way back to the wing. As soon as they entered the double doors, though, all talking ended. They were too interested in what they saw to continue.

Macie was having another shouting match with a staff member. Rozanne didn't recognize the large African-American man that Macie was challenging. "Who's that?" she whispered to Gloria.

"That's Clare," she whispered back. "He's really cool. But I've never seen him so upset before. I wonder what Macie's done now…"

"Get out of my face, you tyrant!" Macie yelled, stamping her foot. "I will not go into that stinky little room again!"

"Now, now Macie…Haven't you had enough of this for one day? Let's just have you go into the room and you can lie down and take a little nap and calm yourself down. Then you can come back out and go to group. How…"

"You creep! I will not go back in there and you can't make me."

"Come on, Macie," Clare replied. "Don't get all worked up. It's better that…."

Macie didn't listen to the rest of his statement. She looked wildly around the hall for an escape route. She spotted the glass door leading to the outside courtyard. She made her decision and ran, full speed into the glass door, cracking the glass partially.

Instantly the area was mass confusion. Macie was rolling around on the floor crying, "My head, oh, my head!" There was a large gash on her forehead, which began spilling blood rapidly down onto the rest of her face.

Clare yelled, "Can I get some help here?"

Gloria sprinted down the hall towards Macie. "Macie! Macie! Are you all right? Oh, Macie, why'd ya have to do it? Why'd ya have to do it?"

Rozanne followed Gloria. This was just too interesting to disregard.

Two staff members emerged that Rozanne didn't recognize. They ran over to Clare and Macie and began administering First Aide to the howling patient.

Clare comforted Macie. "Macie…Macie…Calm down, honey. It'll be all right. We'll get you fixed up and then you can go and lie down and get yourself together, like we talked about, okay? Don't worry Macie. I don't think it's too bad. All head wounds bleed like there's no tomorrow, but the cut is usually not too bad."

As she heard his deep, soothing voice, Macie slowly began to calm down. She quit rolling around and let them bandage her cut. Soon she was sporting a large white bandage on her forehead, which had to be steadied by a gauze wrap around the back of her head. It reminded Rozanne of an oversized baby headband. When the injured patient was repaired, Clare lifted Macie to her feet, put his large, strong arm around her back and led her quietly away.

"Never a dull moment, huh?" said a voice that emerged suddenly from Rozanne's left side. She turned slightly to see Heather, who had moved behind her, unnoticed during all of the commotion.

"What got her so worked up?" Rozanne asked her.

Heather shrugged, "Hard to say. I wasn't there for all of it. I think what really got her going was the phone call she got from her husband. He still wants to cash her check, but refuses to come to see her. He also told her that he'd sold her stereo and CD's. She went bonkers and went down the hall ranting and raving and I guess Clare tried to calm her down, but she wasn't having any part of it. You know Macie."

"Unbelievable," Rozanne said as she stared off into the distance, feeling unnerved by the situation.

Heather interrupted her thoughts. "Hey," she said. "I wanted to ask you something. Do you think you could get me a Book of Mormon?"

"Well…sure. I can't today, but I can have Gary bring one to the hospital tomorrow night. Is that soon enough?" Rozanne was shocked at this turn of events. "Where did this come from?" she wondered to herself.

"Sure. That's fine," Heather said.

"Can I ask you a question now?" Rozanne asked, hesitantly.

"Okay."

"Why do you want one?" Rozanne said. "I didn't even think you were interested in the church. I hope that doesn't offend you."

Heather tilted her head and said, "No, not at all. I'm sort of surprised I want one, too. I've just been thinking about what you said last night. Gloria's had her head buried in the Book of Mormon you gave her all day and so I thought that it wouldn't hurt me to look at one, too."

Gloria nudged Rozanne and said to Heather, "Why don't you try 3rd Nephi first, Heather. You might find that part especially good."

"Okay," Heather agreed. "Will you remind me when I get mine?"

"Sure…sure thing," Rozanne stammered.

After the afternoon groups had ended and the patients were dispersing for free time, the glass door that Macie had cracked when she tried to run away caught Rozanne's eye and she crossed over to it. She could see that the crack had been temporarily repaired with duct tape.

Looking through the unbroken portion of the window, she could see a large courtyard that had a path that wound around in a figure eight. At either end of the circles were cement benches. There was grass all across the courtyard with an occasional small bush or two planted haphazardly in a failed attempt to make the courtyard look cozy. Rozanne could see a man and woman sitting at the far end and the woman looked upset, her arms flailing about her head. They were both too far away from Rozanne to allow her to identify them.

Suddenly, the woman jumped up and stormed away from the man. As she got closer to the door where Rozanne was watching, Rozanne recognized her—it was Laura. She continued to rush away from her husband as fast as her legs could carry her when, abruptly, she stopped and looked straight at Rozanne. As their eyes met through the glass, Rozanne saw something in Laura's eyes that sent a shiver down her spine.

Laura was in misery. Rozanne realized that never before, in her entire life, had she seen a look that was so full of anger and torment. Laura continued to scrutinize Rozanne, almost as if she was silently begging for something—some need that was so deep that there were no words to express it. They both stood fixed, staring at each other like they were stuck in a time continuum.

At last, Laura turned and walked back down the path, past her husband and entered the door of the building at the opposite side of the courtyard. He stood and gazed towards the door, where Rozanne remained, for a brief moment before he sadly turned and followed his wife into the building.

After dinner, Rozanne decided that she would kill some time by watching television in the day room. It would have been a good idea, had circumstances been different, but as it was Halloween that night, she might as well been in the Delta Center during a Jazz game.

The first group to make their appearance was Lizbeth's mother and boyfriend, who had the kids in tow. Lizbeth was right; her kids did look cute. Lizbeth was in her glory. "Look at these guys, Rozanne. Don't they look terrific?" she bragged. "And see what my boyfriend brought me."

She handed Rozanne a greeting card. On the outside was a picture of a baby sitting in a high chair with a bowl of spaghetti poured over the top of its head. When the card was opened it read, "I'm just a mess without you." "Isn't that cute?" Lizbeth gushed. Without waiting for a reply, she snatched the card out of Rozanne's hand and led her family out the door that led to the smoking porch.

Rozanne picked up the remote control off of the table and began scanning the channels to see what was on. Before she had settled on something, Andy, who was escorting his wife and children, came into the room.

"Hi, Rozanne. I'd like you to meet my wife and kids. Tony," Andy said to his son, "this in the lady I was telling you about. She's a music teacher."

"Hi, Tony," Rozanne said, looking towards the boy.

"Tony plays the piano, Rozanne. He has taken lessons for about five years. I think he's pretty good, but I'm probably prejudiced."

"That's nice," she replied. "Who's your teacher, Tony?"

"Mrs. Stanton," the boy shyly told her.

"Do you like her?"

"Yes."

Rozanne looked up at Andy and it didn't take much for him to pick up her message; she didn't want to talk about music teachers. "I'll see you later, okay, Rozanne?"

"Okay," she said, turning back to the television. "Have a nice visit, Andy."

Andy took his wife's hand and led her out of the room and down the hall.

Without giving Rozanne time to breathe, Heather came bounding in the room. "Rozanne! Rozanne! My kids are here! You've got to meet them."

Following Heather was a handsome woman with white hair. She had a little girl, about six years old, by the hand. The child was dressed as Snow White and was carefully carrying a plastic pumpkin full of candy. It was the perfect costume for her. She had deep chestnut-brown hair and had inherited Heather's big, searching eyes.

In close succession came her brothers. The middle boy, who had deep blond hair, appeared to be about eight and was sporting a Superman costume. The older boy was dressed as a pirate and was carrying a sword, which he was enjoying immensely.

"Be careful with that thing, Rusty," instructed Heather. "Rozanne, this are my children; Jessica, Adam and Rusty."

"Jessica, don't you look pretty! What do you have in your pumpkin?" inquired Rozanne.

"Candy. Do you want some?"

"No, thank you. But you are so nice to want to share," Rozanne laughed, amused.

Adam, who had been studying Rozanne, asked, "Why don't you have a costume on? Don't you like Halloween?"

"Sure I do, Adam," Rozanne nodded seriously. "But I guess I forgot to pack one. What do you think I should have dressed up like?"

Adam thought for a minute, "I know. You look like you should be the tooth fairy."

"Adam, don't be so stupid!" declared Rusty.

"Don't worry about it, Rusty," laughed Rozanne. "I think that it would be fun to be the tooth fairy, don't you?"

Heather's mother listened to their conversion uneasily. It was very apparent that she didn't feel that her grandchildren should be talking to a patient. Heather looked apologetically at Rozanne, sighed, and led her family out of the room.

Rozanne turned back to the television. It was Wednesday night. Maybe she could catch a little comedy or something like that…something that could divert her attention from this place for a while. She began watching a show when she heard a noisy group of visitors as they moved down the hall to the day room.

"Hey, Colby man! Where are you bro?"

"Hey Dude, where ya hiding out?"

Laughter…

"Look at that geeky woman over there. Man! Is she a spaz or what?"

Laughter…

"Hey, Colby? Where are all of the freaks?"

At last, Rozanne heard Colby's voice. "Hey dudes, where ya been?"

"Been nowhere, man. You the one that been somewhere. Somewhere not over the rainbow man."

Laughter...

"No kiddin' man. Hey, let's go in here..."

Rozanne heard the group move into the other room. "Thank goodness!" she thought. Her curiosity got the best of her and she snuck over to the doorway to get a peak at Colby and his friends.

There were four young men, about Colby's age and two girls. They were all wearing the same enormous pants that Colby exhibited and were all wearing various shades of blue shirts. Plain blue shirts...

"It figures," muttered Rozanne under her breath. She'd seen kids like that before. They were all over the schools and malls in northern Utah now. The problem was that after a while the normal kids—not realizing that they were imitating gang members—would start wearing the same types of clothing. Then people would think that even good kids looked like they were in gangs. But by then, the gang members usually had moved onto new ways of dressing. It could be confusing to parents, teachers and anyone who dealt with kids.

As she watched Colby and his friends jostling about in the other room, she saw Gloria coming towards her. "Hi!" said Gloria. "What are you doing?".

Rozanne turned back to the day room and to her chair. "I was trying to watch some TV, but this place is too noisy tonight."

"I know what you mean," Gloria agreed, sitting down next to her. "I think everyone has visitors tonight."

"Not me," lamented Rozanne.

"Me, either."

Rozanne thought about that. Gloria never had any visitors. Gloria never got any phone calls. What was she going to do when she got out of here? But Gloria had something else on her mind. She brightened and said happily, "Hey, I've been reading the Book of Mormon today."

"I noticed," Rozanne told her. "How is it going?"

"Good," Gloria said. "I haven't read it since I got home from my mission. Stupid of me, I guess. But I just got so mixed up with everything that was going on."

Rozanne didn't reply, but just waited for Gloria to continue. They sat in silence for a while before Gloria spoke again. "Rozanne, I've been reading in the book of Alma. He says that Christ went forth suffering pains and afflictions and temptations of every kind so that he can take upon him our pains and sicknesses. Do you think that means that Christ knows how we feel? After all, he never suffered a major depression or was mentally ill or anything like that. Do you think he truly knows how we feel?"

Rozanne had never considered this question before. She wondered if she could answer Gloria's query adequately. But as she spoke, knowledge she had gained from years of scripture study returned to her memory. "I know that in the Doctrine and Covenants we are taught that he descended below all things so that he could understand all things. I think it probably happened while he was in the Garden of Gethsemane. We don't totally understand what he went through while he was there. It must have been awful. He bled from every pore and an angel even came and helped him out. It must have been so terrible that it would have killed an ordinary person. Maybe during this time he felt some of the feelings we feel when we are discouraged and depressed, and so he understands how we feel."

"I never thought of that before," said Gloria. "That makes sense. How did you come up with that idea?"

"I'm not sure," Rozanne answered. "It was probably just years of learning about things. I remember something else, too. Alma the Younger had reason to know Christ understood these kinds of feelings."

"He did?" Gloria said.

Rozanne nodded at her. "Do you remember how bad he was before he repented? He was out teaching people that the church wasn't true. He was trying to destroy the church. When the angel visited him and called him to repentance, he realized how terrible he was and he fainted and was in a coma for three days. He must have really suffered because he said that he wished he could disappear. I know how that feels…to want to disappear…"

"I do, too," Gloria said.

Rozanne looked at Gloria. Maybe she had been more depressed than Rozanne had realized. Rozanne grimaced in sympathy and continued, "Anyway, Alma felt so bad about what he had done. Then, when he remembered what his father had taught him about Christ, he called out in his mind for Christ's help. Immediately, he felt such joy! He had never felt so happy before. It was quite a contrast to the misery he had been in. Christ must have known how to help him for Alma to become so suddenly changed."

Gloria looked out of the window for a long time after Rozanne had finished. Rozanne didn't feel like talking either. "I hadn't thought of that before," she thought to herself. "I hadn't thought of that before. Christ knows how I feel and he understands. He still loves me." A warm feeling passed through her and she felt more hope than she had known in a long, long time.

"You loser! You creep! What's the matter with you? You promised me that you'd come here tonight…No, I don't care about that…No…There is no way on this earth I am going to let you cash that check, especially now. Well, forget about it then; just forget about it…BANG!!"

Gloria and Rozanne looked at each other. It was Macie.

Gloria jumped up. "I better go. You never know what will happen. Maybe I can stop her." She ran out of the room and Rozanne could hear her as she tried to calm Macie down,

"Macie, what's going on?"

"That creep I'm married to…He said he was going to come tonight. He promised me that he'd come tonight. I waited and waited and waited in my room, but he never came. He never came." Macie started to cry.

"Come on, Macie," soothed Gloria. "Let's go down to my room for a while, okay?"

"Okay," sniffed Macie through her tears.

Rozanne could hear Macie crying as Gloria took her down the hall. "This is too depressing, "she thought. She felt a pain growing in her right temple that made her feel like her head was going to explode. She got up and went to the staff window. Clare was behind the desk with his back to her. It looked like he was writing in some charts. Rozanne waited a minute, but when he didn't turn around she knocked on the window.

"Hey, Clare!"

Clare turned around and saw her. His eyebrows knit together with concern when he saw the expression on her face. "What's up?"

"I have a terrible headache," she moaned. "Can I get something for it?"

"Just a minute. I'll look in your chart and see what the doc has ordered for you." Clare reached over to the hanging file rack and pulled out a chart. After he flipped through the pages he said, "I don't see anything here for you."

Rozanne didn't say anything. She just felt like crying. "Why am I so upset?" she thought. "This deal with Macie isn't anything new."

Clare studied her for a minute before he spoke, "Are you okay? Do you feel safe?"

"Yes. That's not a problem. I guess Macie just got to me. I don't understand how someone could be newly married and not care enough about his wife to come and see her in the hospital. As I began to think about it, my head started to ache."

"Why don't you try this?" Clare suggested. Go in and get yourself some juice or something and then go to your room and lie down for a while. I'll call your doctor and ask him if I can give you some Advil or Tylenol. Then I'll come and get you."

"Thanks, I'll try that." Rozanne replied, turning to go to her room. "I've never seen so many sad, sad people," she thought. "I guess I was too sheltered. It makes me feel like an idiot being here. I should have been able to handle my problems better. I should have...Why am I such a mess? My life isn't that bad...No, not bad at all...Oh, I'm such a jerk. I've just caused too many problems for too many people...I should have been able to handle it...I've just ruined everything..."

As she continued down the hall, she began to feel herself slipping over the edge of a psychological cliff. By the time she got to her room, she just wanted to curl up in a ball and climb back into a dark closet somewhere.

She entered her room without turning on the lights and was relieved to see that Laura wasn't there. She was alone. She threw herself down on the bed and began to sob. "I wish I could disappear...No, not really disappear...just go back in time."

She tried to think of a time that she'd like to experience again. There was the period of time when they were in California. That wasn't too bad. "We should have never moved back to Utah. It's all my fault. We should have never moved back...But wait a minute, we would have had to move anyway because of Gary's job..."

Rozanne rubbed her temples, "I know...How about when we in Oklahoma? Yes, that was a good time...I loved being in college...That was a very happy time...But wait a minute...I didn't have my two youngest children yet and I wouldn't wish them away for anything...Oh, rats...I can't do this to myself anymore...I've got to stop this!"

Rozanne jumped up and rushed out of the room. As she was barreling up the hall she bumped into Macie. "Hold on," Macie demanded. "Where do you think you're going so fast?"

"Nowhere...nowhere..." Rozanne answered.

Macie squinted at her. She decided to forgive Rozanne. She reached out and grabbed Rozanne's arm, preventing her from slipping away. Then she looked around the hallway to see if they were alone. When she was satisfied that they were, she whispered, "Rozanne, look at this. I want to show you something." Holding out her left arm, she pushed up her sleeve and displayed her wrist.

Rozanne couldn't see anything unusual about the wrist, but understood that Macie wanted her to notice something about it. She looked closer and asked, "Just what am I supposed to be seeing?"

Macie snorted indignantly. "Can't you tell? I tried to slit my wrist a few minutes ago. But it didn't work out because I used a plastic knife. They don't work very well."

Rozanne squinted her eyes and studied Macie's arm a little harder. Yes, there was a slight indentation, sort of like a scratch that you would make with a short fingernail. It was about three inches long right along the base of her wrist. It was so light that it was hard to see. "Why did you try to do that?" Rozanne asked.

Macie thrust her chin out proudly. "I just got so mad at my husband that I wanted to get even with him...so...I tried to cut myself," she bragged.

"You idiot! Why did you do that?" Rozanne jumped at the sound of Heather's voice coming from behind her. She turned and looked at Heather. She was glaring at Macie with such vehemence and disgust, that it made Rozanne shiver. "Macie, you just make me sick. How could you pretend to do something like that?"

"Shows you what you know, Heather," Macie insisted. "I wasn't pretending nothin'. I wanted to kill myself."

Heather gave Macie a dirty look. "You did not! You just wanted some attention—that's all. Nobody tries to slit their wrist with a plastic knife if they're serious. You idiot! Now they're going to make your life miserable. Macie, you better watch out or they're going to send you to the state hospital. You don't want to go there. I've heard stories about that place. If you'd just start trying to do something for yourself, maybe you could get better and get on with your life. But no, you have to try to cut yourself with a plastic knife, of all things!"

Heather glowered at Macie for a minute longer before storming down the hall to the staff window. She started banging on the window, "Hey, is somebody there? You've got to do something with Macie before she really does something crazy!"

Clare slid open the window and Heather told him what had happened. Immediately, the door to the right of the staff window opened and Clare strode out down the hall towards Macie. Macie looked wildly around her surroundings for a minute before she made her move. She tore off down the hall away from Clare. With long, fast strides Clare quickly caught up with her and grabbed her by the arm. "Macie, what's wrong with you? Why won't you let us help you?"

"Get out of my face!"

"Come on Macie," Clare demanded. "You know what this means. Dr. Manning warned you that if you had anymore trouble you would be on twenty-four hour watch. So, let's get started. Let's go into your room and get your things and we'll move you down to isolation and pick out a room."

Macie glowered darkly at him and stamped on his foot. "I told you to get out of my face," she said with a hard, angry voice.

Clare used his large presence to force her to back up against the wall. "Macie, we can do this the easy way or the hard way. What's it going to be?"

Macie slid down the wall that Clare had pinned her against. Once she hit the floor she bent over and buried her face in her lap.

"Macie, I'm waiting."

There was a long pause before Macie finally answered. "Oh, all right. I'm coming."

Clare helped her up and they walked back up the hall and disappeared into Macie's room.

"She's really something, isn't she?" asked Heather.

"I guess so," Rozanne replied.

Heather studied Rozanne's profile. "Why don't we go into the group room and color? You look like you need to calm down."

As they walked, Rozanne wondered about Heather. She was so deeply troubled and yet, she seemed to be the most take-charge person Rozanne had ever known. At times, she could seem so vulnerable, and then other times, she seemed so strong. Heather always seemed to know what to do to help the other patients out—sometimes even more than the hospital's staff. It was puzzling.

Heather settled Rozanne at the table with a new picture and was helping her sharpen the colored pencils when Tawny burst into the room, "Guess what? Guess what? I'm going home! Oh, I'm going home!"

Heather and Rozanne exchanged shocked looks. Tawny going home? She had practically been comatose the day before! Heather asked, "Tawny how could this happen?"

"Dr. Morrison said that he has just been waiting for me to take an interest in myself. It was that simple! When I started eating and talking, he decided to let me go home! Can you believe it? My mom is down in the office checking me out right now. I get to go home! I just can't believe it!"

Tawny immediately disappeared back out of the door. She was only gone a short time when she reappeared, escorted by an elderly woman who was carrying an infant dressed in a blue, fuzzy bunting suit.

"Heather…Rozanne…this is my mom. And this…this is my son!" Tawny squealed, grabbing the baby from her mother and hugging him tight. The baby looked over his mother's shoulder at the two women. He was only about three months old.

Suddenly an idea popped into Rozanne's head; Tawny probably had been suffering from Postpartum Depression. "Tawny, I hope everything is going to be all right for you from now on," she said.

"Oh, I just know it is," Tawny said happily, hugging her son tightly. "I'm on medication now and I'll keep going to Dr. Morrison until I get totally better. But the best part is I can go home! I need to be with my son, I know that now, don't I?" Tawny looked at her mother and smiled brightly. Her mother put her arm around Tawny's waist and they left the room.

Heather and Rozanne watched as they walked down the hall, pushed the button to be let out of the wing and then disappeared forever as the big double doors closed behind them. There was total silence for several minutes before the quiet was broken by the sound of Heather's black colored pencil moving quickly back and forth, back and forth across her page.

Day 4

▼

Rozanne sat on her bed, chewing on the end of her pencil. It would soon be time for morning group, but she wanted to write in her journal. Even though her mind was whirling, she managed to write, "I'm scared and upset today. If I don't go back to teaching school we won't be able to pay the rent and we'll have to move. The kids are finally all happy and doing well in school. I can't do this to them. What can I do about this situation?"

She began making a list of their bills. Then she subtracted them from what Gary made. It didn't add up—she was going to have to work. Their rent was so high…They had tried to find a more reasonable place to live, but that was a hard thing to do in the Salt Lake Valley. "There just isn't anyway out of this mess," she thought. "I better do something else before I get upset."

Rozanne was just starting the list of her priorities, as Dr. Beall had suggested, when she heard a knock on the door. It was Mattie. "Rozanne, it is time for group. Are you coming?"

"Yes. I'll be right there." Rozanne sprung to her feet, carrying her journal with her as she walked up the hall. "I'll finish that later," she thought. "There's still a lot to do."

Rozanne noticed immediately that Macie wasn't with other patients as she entered the group room. She went to the table where Heather was coloring and sat down next to her. "Where's Macie?" she whispered.

"Didn't you hear?" Heather whispered back. "Macie freaked out on them again last night and they had to give her some heavy-duty medications to calm her down. I think she's probably sleeping it off. I'm getting worried about her. She seems to be going down hill."

Rozanne felt her stomach clench. It terrified her that someone could actually get worse in the hospital. "I thought we are supposed to get better here—or at least begin to get better. I wonder if there is anything that I can do to help Macie…No, that's ridiculous! I'm in no position to be helping anybody right now."

"Rozanne…Rozanne." she heard.

"Huh? What? Oh, sorry…"

"Are you all right?" asked Rhaun. "I asked you a question, but you seemed to be far away."

Rozanne looked up at him and let her eyes focus on his face. She knew the other patients were waiting. "I know" she answered. "Sorry…What did you want to know?"

"Did you write down the list of tapes in your head, like I asked you to?" he asked.

"Actually, I had already completed it when you suggested it to me yesterday."

"Have you thought anything about the list since you wrote it down?" Rhaun continued.

"No…I guess I haven't."

"I see that you have your journal with you," he continued. "I was wondering if you would look at your list and see if there is an irrational idea on it that we could use as an example, as we continue our discussion from yesterday. Do you remember that we were going to talk about how to get rid of irrational ideas?"

"Yes, I remember. Okay, that sounds good." She opened her journal and looked at the list. There were several choices that she felt were possibilities. She began to read, "Don't cry. Don't get mad. Don't talk back. Mothers take the smallest piece. Children come first…"

"Whoa!" Rhaun exclaimed, holding up his hand to stop her. "That's too many! How many more of those do you have on that list of yours?"

"A few…"

Rhaun turned to the group and said, "Why don't we help Rozanne out? Which of the ideas she read would you like to use?"

"Don't get mad," said Howard.

"Don't cry," said Gloria.

"Don't talk back, "said Andy.

"Oh-oh," said Rhaun. "Can we possibly come to an agreement? Rozanne, which one do you like the best?"

Rozanne pulled a face. She didn't like any of them. "I'm not sure," she replied.

"Which one makes your stomach clench up when you think about it?"

She knew the answer immediately. "Don't talk back."

"Why did you choose that one?" he asked.

Rozanne felt embarrassed to answer his question. She knew what the response would be. "Because I feel guilty when I talk back to people."

Rhaun smiled, "Why doesn't that surprise me? Let's use that one. Is that all right with everybody?"

No one objected, so Rhaun moved on. "Let's make a list of reasons we don't like to talk back. Rozanne has given us the first one." Rhaun wrote, "Makes me feel guilty" on the white board. "Anyone else?"

"I know," answered Andy, "how about fear? I don't talk back because I am afraid of what will happen to me if I do."

"Good," Rhaun said. "What else?"

"I don't feel that I'm smart enough. I think I don't deserve to talk back to someone. It's easier just to go along." stammered Gloria.

"Excellent!" Rhaun exclaimed, as he wrote "self-doubt" with a red marker under Andy's response.

"It doesn't do any good to talk back to people," said Heather. "The fact is that most people don't care what you think about things."

"Do you really believe that?" asked Rhaun.

"Yes, I do," Heather answered.

"I'll tell you what I think," smirked Colby. "You people are the biggest group of losers I've ever seen. Afraid to talk back…Ha! There ain't nothin' to it, man. I don't care what nobody says. I do what I do. Ain't nobody going to tell me nothin'. You're all wimps!"

"Colby," Rhaun said. "I hear what you're saying, but I've got to tell you, you're just plain wrong. Your irrational thought pattern is just the opposite of Rozanne's. She's too sensitive of other people's opinions of her and you're not sensitive enough. Now, do you have anything else to add to the discussion? Something that could be helpful?"

"No, man. Don't worry. You'll be hearin' nothin' else from me today." Colby threatened as he stood, gesturing angrily at Rhaun, and swaggered out of the room, holding his pants up with his left hand as he went.

After Colby had disappeared, Rhaun turned to the group and said, "Shall we go on? Rozanne, why don't you think of a time when you wanted to talk back, but you didn't do it. Then we'll discuss it."

It was Rozanne's first teaching assignment in Utah. She was the new orchestra teacher in a very nice, middle-class junior high school. Rozanne liked the school a lot, but she had a terrible problem; she didn't get along with the band teacher. Rozanne wasn't quite sure why. She kept trying to get along with the other teacher, but the band teacher wasn't having any part of it

It seemed like everything Rozanne did was an irritant to the other teacher. Rozanne shouldn't write on the board in the room. Rozanne shouldn't hang posters up on the wall. Rozanne's students didn't put the stands away in neat little lines with their feet crossed and the tops down every single time. Rozanne forgot to turn off the stereo. The list of Rozanne's failings seemed to extend forever into the vast universe…

Finally, the principal talked to Rozanne about the disagreements.

"I don't know what to do about it," Rozanne lamented to the principal. "Tell me what you want me to do and I'll do it. I just want to get along. I've never had this problem with another teacher before!" But the principal was unable to give her useful solutions and the problem continued.

One day, Rozanne got an idea. "I know! I'll surprise the band teacher with balloons and give her a card. Maybe we could just let bygones be bygones and start again!" She went to the local grocery store and selected a huge bouquet of brightly colored helium balloons and a humorous card to be delivered to the band teacher on one of the teacher workdays.

It didn't work. The band teacher never even acknowledged the receipt of the balloons.

Life continued—rather uncomfortably for Rozanne—but still, it continued. Then one day it happened—the disaster…

It was February. February was their recruiting month. The school counselors arranged for the incoming 7th graders to be bused to the school for an assembly that introduced them to middle school programs. The band, choir, and orchestra would play for the students. Representatives from each group would then talk to the students about the benefits of being in their programs.

The choir sang. Some of the choir students spoke to the new 7th graders. The band played. Some of the band kids spoke to the group. The orchestra played. Some of the orchestra students talked to the new 7th graders.

Rozanne didn't realize it, but one of the orchestra students she had selected to speak for their group was a loose cannon and the foolish, young girl made a remark that made it seem far superior to be in the orchestra. Rozanne knew just was just being over-enthusiastic, but the remark made Rozanne feel very uneasy.

Nevertheless, Rozanne understood her student's enthusiasm. She had worked very hard to build this feeling in the group. Before this year, the orchestra students were looked on as the "dregs" of middle school society. Now they felt proud to be in the orchestra. This new pride had simply bubbled to the surface. Rozanne crossed her fingers and hoped for the best.

Two hours after the assembly had concluded, she heard a knock on her classroom's door. She was teaching a group of General Music students, so she told them to look at their theory pages and she'd be right back. She opened the door and stepped outside. The band teacher stood in the hallway, her arms crossed angrily. The choir teacher shadowed her in a show of solidarity.

"Just where do you get off pulling a stunt like that?" the band teacher demanded.

"What stunt?" Rozanne asked, her face growing hot.

"Coaching your kids to make band and choir seem stupid. Just who do you think you are? I've had enough of you. You've had it. Don't you think for a minute you are getting away with this..."

Rozanne panicked. She hadn't put that kid up to it. Before the assembly she had gone over with the students what they were going to say and it was totally innocent. The overly enthusiastic girl had simply gotten carried away.

As she listened to the tirade, Rozanne felt her heart pound and the vein in her right temple growing tighter and tighter until she felt like it was going to explode. Every now and then she would attempt to talk. "But..." or "Wait..." she'd try to say, but the band teacher wasn't in a mood to listen to her. It would take a force of equal caliber to stop her.

The biggest problem was this: Rozanne began to self-talk to herself as the blustering went on, "I really am a jerk! I should have known this would happen. I should have realized that she would be so mad and try to head her off. I shouldn't have let that student talk. I should have known she would get carried away. Oh, nothing ever works out for me. Now I'm going to have to transfer away from this school and I love the kids so much here that it's going to kill me. If I try to defend myself it will just make things worse. I've got to be patient and not let her get to me. She just hates me, that's all. Nothing can ever be right here at this school again. Oh, this all happened because we left California...We should have stayed there...but we had to leave, didn't we?

You see, nothing ever goes right for me…"

She continued to beat herself up as the band teacher persisted with her unrelenting outburst. Soon Rozanne began to feel herself slipping away. She felt like she was just to the edge of her endurance when suddenly, she looked down the hall and spotted the principal accompanied by the vice-principal and one of the school counselors. Rozanne motioned to them with a desperate look on her face and they made their way to her side. The three of them managed to calm the band teacher down and get her and the choir teacher (who never did say too much) to leave.

Rozanne started to hyperventilate, "I'm going to have to quit," she muttered. "I'm going to have to quit. I can't take this anymore." The principal got a concerned look on her face and assured Rozanne that things would change. This episode had shown her quite clearly what the true situation was. She assured Rozanne that she would speak to the band teacher about the incident.

"Tell her that she can't talk to me anymore!" Rozanne pleaded. "Please, tell her that. She can send me notes in my box or messages through you, but I can't take this anymore."

The principal agreed. The band teacher was not to talk to Rozanne again for the rest of the school year. It was no surprise to anyone when Rozanne transferred at the end of the year to another school. The band teacher had won.

"That's a good example. We can use several elements of it," remarked Rhaun. "Let's look at how you could have handled the situation better. First, in order to analyze what happened, you should write down the facts of the situation. Only include the objective facts, not the way you felt about what happened."

"Should I stick just to the recruiting situation?" Rozanne asked him.

Rhaun nodded as he raised his eyebrows. "That's enough for now, don't you think?"

"I guess so!" piped in Lizbeth. "What a jerk!"

Rozanne looked over at Lizbeth and smiled. It felt good to have someone take her side. Turning her attention back to the question at hand, she remarked, "I think I can do that. First, we were at a recruiting event and all three groups had to play for the new kids. Then each group got to tell the incoming seventh graders about the benefits of joining their organization. One of my students got carried away and said too much. This made the band teacher angry and she yelled at me. I panicked and started to say irrational things to myself."

"Good," Rhaun said, as he sketched a brief list of the events on the board. Looking back over his shoulder at Rozanne he instructed, "Now let's list some of your irrational self-talk."

Rozanne grimaced. That would be harder to do. "How about this," she said, "nothing ever works out for me."

"Yes," motivated Rhaun. "That's right. Can you think of another one?"

Rozanne tried to remember. Then she thought of a statement that she told herself on a regular basis. "Rhaun," she asked skeptically, "I think I may have another one. Wasn't it irrational when I told myself that it happened because we left California?"

"That's right," he assured her. "You can't blame your move from California for your current difficulties. Anything else?"

"I don't know," she hesitated.

"I know one!" said Howard. "Rozanne, you couldn't have known before hand that it was going to happen. That's just not logical."

"How about when you said that you would have to transfer away? You didn't have to transfer. You chose to transfer," added Heather.

The group murmured their approval of Heather's remark. Andy raised his hand to get their attention. "When you said that if you would defend yourself it would make things worse," he stated, "that wasn't necessarily true. Maybe if you had defended yourself earlier none of this would have happened,"

"I don't know," replied Rozanne. "She didn't seem willing to listen to me."

"I think I heard one," said Lizbeth. "You said you're a jerk. That sure sounds irrational to me to make that kind of self-judgement."

"Why is that, Lizbeth? Didn't you just call that band teacher a jerk?" asked Howard.

"But that was different," she retorted. "Rozanne shouldn't be calling herself a jerk."

"You're all correct," answered Rhaun. "Rozanne, you were a hotbed of irrational ideas that day. I bet that this is a problem for you. You might want to think some more about it."

"You're probably right," she agreed. "But what do I do about it?"

"Let's go on to the next steps and maybe you'll figure that out," Rhaun told her as he turned back to the white board. "After you write down the irrational self-talk, you should focus on your emotional responses to the situation. Rozanne, can you make a one or two word label for how you felt that day?"

Rozanne closed her eyes and tried to remember how she felt when the band teacher was yelling at her. She managed to recall the angry look on the band teacher's face. She opened her eyes and said, "I felt misunderstood, embarrassed, and worthless."

Rhaun nodded his endorsement. "Sounds about right," he said as he wrote what she had said on the board. "Now that you've identified the emotions you experienced, you're ready to begin talking back to yourself in better ways."

"How do you do that?" asked Heather. "I think I just stop at labeling my emotions. It's hard to know what to do after that."

"Not me," said Lizbeth. "Sometimes I enjoy getting mad at people."

"If you enjoy it so, much how come you're in here?" asked Howard.

Lizbeth tossed her head impatiently, as she threw Howard the only comeback she could think of, "Never you mind!"

"Okay Rhaun, go on." said Heather.

"First, you select one of the ideas that isn't rational. Let's work on this one," Rhaun said as he pointed to the statement on the board, *Nothing ever works out for me.* "Now group let's decide," he said. "Are there any facts that support this idea?"

"No way!" said Heather. "Rozanne, don't you have a great husband and four kids that are alive and well? It seems to me that something very important has worked out for you."

"You have a college degree, don't you?" said Gloria. "I'd like to have one of those."

"All right. All right," interrupted Rozanne, impatiently. "I get the point. Rhaun, what's next?"

"Next, you move on to discover what evidence there is that refutes the false idea. Heather and Gloria have already mentioned a few facts. You have a nice family and a college degree. Can you think of anything else?"

"I've had more positive than negative teaching experiences," Rozanne said. "That shows that it's not true."

"Good, you've got the jest of it," Rhaun replied. "Now that you understand that phase of the process, we'll move on. Are you ready?" he said, looking around the room for consensus. When he saw that he had it, he continued his discourse. "The next step is to decide if there is any evidence that suggests that the statement you are working with is true." Pointing at the statement, *"Nothing ever works out for me"* again, he looked at Rozanne and asked, "What do you think? Can you think of any evidence that suggests that you never succeed?"

"No, I guess it's not true at all," Rozanne returned. "I've had plenty of successes. It just feels like I'm a failure at everything during a crisis. Maybe I need to stop saying that to myself. All right, Rhaun," she sighed, "I get it. What's next?"

"You decide what's the worst thing that could happen to you because of the event," answered Rhaun.

"Oh, I like that!" said Gloria. "I think that could be very helpful to me. Maybe if I could think of the worst thing that would happen, I wouldn't be so afraid of everything."

Rozanne looked at Gloria and moaned, "The worst thing that could happen to me, did happen. I transferred. I should have been tougher and stuck it out at that school. I really liked it there, except for my relationship with the band teacher, of course. I loved the kids, the facilities, the area, and my classes. I had friends on the faculty. I let the band teacher run me out of there because of my own insecurities and as a result, I got myself into a situation that was much worse and now here I am!"

"Think, Rozanne, think! Was that really the worst thing that could have happened?" insisted Rhaun.

"I don't know," she groaned. "I'm having a hard time being objective. I really wish I wouldn't have transferred. It was such a big mistake."

"Rozanne," said Andy. "What if the principal sided with the band teacher and you were fired. Wouldn't that have been the worst thing that could have happened to you that day?"

"Oh, but that wouldn't have happened," Rozanne insisted. "The principal would have had to prove that I was a bad teacher to be able to fire me. Besides, even though she was the band teacher's friend, the principal was very nice to me. She really tried to be fair. It wasn't her fault. I don't hold her responsible."

Rozanne opened her journal and fiercely began drawing jagged boxes around a blank page. She felt so annoyed with herself. " I guess the worst thing that could have happened was that I could have gotten so upset that I could have walked out of there that day and quit my job. That would have been awful! I would have beat myself up about that the rest of my life. I'm glad I wasn't that stupid."

"So the worst thing didn't happen," said Rhaun. "That's good, isn't it? Now that you realize this you can move on. After you have considered what would have been the worst thing that could have happened to you, you turn it completely around and try to think about what good things might happen to you because of the incident,"

"What good things?" Rozanne said. "It seems to me that this event was a turning point in my life. It just led to a lot of trouble."

"I can understand that," Rhaun said, "but how about this? You might have learned that it was important to develop better coping skills. You might have learned that it was important to learn to deal with angry people better. You might have learned that it doesn't help to stand there and let someone beat up on you. Did you learn any of those things?"

"Yes. I did learn those things. I just didn't know it at the time and I still don't know how to do any of it," sighed Rozanne.

"Give it some time, Rozanne," said Andy. "You needed help to learn these things. Now you're on your way."

Rozanne looked up at Andy. "It's funny you say that. I got to be quite good friends with the counselor after that. He told me that I should get some help learning to be more assertive. He told me that I should have just put my hands on my hips and told the band teacher to grow up. I guess he was right, after all."

"It sounds like you are already getting some ideas, Rozanne," said Lizbeth. "This is so interesting to me. I think I do the same thing. I just stand there and let people yell at me without standing up for myself."

"Me, too," said Gloria.

"I do it, too sometimes," said Andy.

"I'm not surprised that many of you have problems with this, to some degree," said Rhaun. "People that are depressed or have substance abuse problems aren't that different. They just use diverse methods to deal with the frustrations they're experiencing. Rozanne's frustrations went underground and eventually she broke under the stress."

"I drink...or I used to drink," said Andy. "I'm off of that now—for good, I hope!"

"Is that all, Rhaun?" asked Howard.

Rhaun looked at Howard and shook his head. "No. You still need to learn to do one more thing—and this is the most important step. You need to learn to substitute better self-talk for irrational ideas when you get into these situations. For example, during the period of time when the band teacher was yelling at Rozanne, she could have told herself that she is strong. She's lived through hard times before and she can live through this. She could have told herself that it is better to face difficult situations that run away from them. She could have told herself that she has succeeded before and she can succeed again. These positive thoughts would have helped her cope with the stressful situation. They would have given her the strength she needed at the time to deal with it."

"I get it," said Rozanne, "but it sounds too easy. I have a feeling that it isn't easy at all."

"You're right about that, Rozanne," Rhaun replied. "It's not easy to learn new thought patterns and responses to situations. It's not easy, but it *is* possible. Here's some homework for each of you. I'm giving you some worksheets that have all of the elements I've listed on them."

Rhaun held up a book for the group. "I got it out of this book called *The Relaxation & Stress Reduction Workbook*. It was put together by Martha Davis, Elizabeth Robbins Eshelmean, and Matthew McKay and I highly recommend it. Here, I'll pass it around the room for you to look at."

Rhaun handed the book and the stack of worksheets to Howard. "If you'll try filling of the worksheets out everyday as you deal with stressful situations, you'll begin to understand your thought processes better. If you use them and you still have problems with irrational thoughts, there are probably some things that are making it hard for you to change."

"Like what?" asked Heather.

"Like you still don't believe that your thoughts cause emotions," he told her." "Like your self-talk comes so quickly that you have difficulty catching it. Keep a journal and write down what you can catch or carry around one of those little 'clickers' that athletes use to count the number of times you catch yourself thinking irrational things. Rozanne, you could count the number of times you feel guilty."

"She'd wear one out," laughed Lizbeth.

"Oh, we shouldn't tease you about it," said Rhaun when he saw Rozanne's red cheeks. "Some guilt is important, very important. It helps us to know when we need to change. You seem to have gone over the edge with guilt, though, Rozanne. You need to learn to tell the difference between healthy guilt and unhealthy guilt, if that makes sense."

"Yes. It does," Rozanne sighed. "Where can you buy those things—those clickers?"

Rhaun thought briefly. "I think you might try a good sporting goods store," he replied.

When they had finished, the patients wandered out in the hall for a break. Rozanne decided to go into the day room and see if she could catch a little of the Rosie O'Donnell show on TV. It was about time for it to start. Instead, Macie headed her off. "I was looking for you."

"Me? Why me?" Rozanne said. She certainly didn't want to talk to Macie right now. She was tired. Group had been long and difficult for her and she wanted to zone out in front of the television set for a while. Macie didn't let Rozanne's obvious annoyance phase her a bit. "I wanted to talk to you about something," she insisted, grabbing at Rozanne's arm. "I want you to come with me."

"Go with you? Where?" asked Rozanne.

"In here," replied Macie, pointing at the room leading into the staff room. Then she pounded on it and yelled, "Hey, Mattie. Let me in, will ya?"

Mattie opened the door and asked, "What do you want, Macie?"

"I want Rozanne to come in with me and see my room," she asked innocently. "Is that okay?"

"That would be fine." Mattie opened the door and Macie succeeded in gripping Rozanne's arm too firmly to allow her to escape and hurriedly pushed her through the open doorway.

Once they were inside, Rozanne realized that the area was larger than it appeared from the patient's side of the window. There were several doorways that she hadn't noticed before. One led to a supply room and one led to a room that could be a conference area. There were also two doors that remained closed. "I wonder what's in there," she thought.

"Look! Here's my room," Macie said. "I can't have much in here. They're afraid of what I'll do, but they let me keep these." Macie pulled her into the middle of the room and pointed to the windowsill, where she had propped up a small picture of the Salt Lake temple and the Book of Mormon Rozanne had given her.

"They look out of place here, somehow," Rozanne thought as she said to Macie, "Oh, good. I'm glad you still have the Book of Mormon. Where did you get the picture of the temple?"

"My visiting teachers came here once; they brought it to me," answered Macie. "They only came one time, but it was nice."

Macie's speech about Visiting Teachers reminded Rozanne of something she was curious about. "Macie," she asked, "didn't I hear you say that you went on a mission? Tell me about it."

Macie's face lit up. "I went to the Toronto, Ontario mission. It was cold up there. I got to see Niagara Falls. Did you know that it rains ice up there in the winter? It gets hard to walk around."

"How long were you there?" asked Rozanne.

"Oh, I get it," Macie retorted, offended. "You want to know if I finished my mission."

"No," Rozanne quickly said, "that's not what I meant at all. I wanted to know how long you were in Niagara Falls. My husband went to that mission, too. He loved Niagara Falls."

Macie relaxed. "Just a little while…that was before the president sent me home."

"Sent you home?" Rozanne repeated.

"Yeah," Macie said, shrugging her shoulders to indicate feigned indifference. "I came home early. I had been out about ten months. I kept getting depressed. It was hard to go out and do the work. It was harder on my companions. The mission president kept trying to help me, but finally, he decided that I had better come home and get some professional help."

"How long ago was that?" Rozanne inquired carefully.

Macie rubbed her nose. "I don't know…maybe about a year ago or so. I was older when I went on my mission to begin with."

They sat and looked awkwardly at each other. Macie obviously wanted something, but wasn't ready to divulge her secret yet. Rozanne decided to discuss another topic that interested her. "How long did you know your husband before you got married to him?" she asked.

"Six weeks," Macie replied, preoccupied with her own thoughts.

"Six weeks?"

"Yeah," Macie shrugged, unconcerned. "I only dated him about two weeks, though. We suddenly decided to get married and so we drove out to Reno, Nevada and did it. One day I wasn't married and the next day I was. He moved into my apartment. I thought I would be happier when I got married, but everything just got worse. I think he doesn't love me at all. I've been so stupid."

Rozanne began to feel sorry for Macie. "What are you going to do?" she asked.

"I don't know. I know Heather doesn't think I understand what's going on, but I do. I just can't deal with it. I get so mad at him and then I want to do something—anything—just to get back at him. I wish I could just die."

Macie and Rozanne sat, side by side, on the bed and looked out of the window. Rozanne noticed that the window had a metal screen, sort of like chicken wire, imbedded into the glass. Macie didn't say anything so Rozanne took the opportunity to examine the room thoroughly.

It was tiny. Just a bed, bolted to the floor, that had some sheets, a pillow and one blanket on it. There was also a small shelf that was bolted to the painted cinder-block wall behind it. It served as a nightstand. The room didn't have a closet or chairs. Rozanne decided that the worst thing about being in this room was the window in the door. Macie would not be allowed any privacy. Rozanne guessed that the window was placed there so that staff could keep an eye on the occupant at all times.

Macie broke into her thoughts, "Rozanne I wanted to ask you a question. That's why I brought you in here."

"Okay," Rozanne answered. "What do you want to know?"

Macie bounced her leg and reached up and ran her fingers through her hair. She stopped moving. Then she wrung her hands in despair and looked hopefully at Rozanne. "Do you really," she began. "I mean, do you absolutely believe that God loves everybody?"

Rozanne was surprised by the question, but answered, "Sure, Macie. I believe that."

"Even somebody like me?" Macie insisted, thumping her chest agitatedly.

"What do you mean by that?" Rozanne returned.

The leg started bouncing again. "Could he love somebody as messed up as me?" Macie looked wildly around the room. Jumping suddenly to her feet, she began to pace the small area nervously. "I mean," she agonized, "I came home from my mission early. I'm a freak. I should have been able to do it…I'm fat…I'm ugly…My parents don't love me…I don't have any skills…I'm on Social Security, you know, because of my depression. It's bad. I'm worse than most of you are, I think. The doctors even helped me become declared disabled by the government. My Social Security check is the one that my husband wants to cash so bad. Now, to make things worse, I've married a complete loser. I knew better at the time, but he was the only guy to ever pay me any attention and it felt good, for a little while, anyway." Macie stopped launching herself about the room and faced Rozanne. "How could God love someone like me anymore?"

Rozanne swallowed. This was going to be hard. She felt overwhelmed by everything Macie said, but she did believe that Heavenly Father loved Macie. She believed Heavenly Father loved all of his children. That's what was keeping Rozanne alive.

"Mommy! Mommy! Can I get in your bed? I'm scared!"
"Go back to bed," Father grumbled.
"But I'm scared, Mama!" pleaded Rozanne.
"I'll take care of her," Mother said, as she stood and reached for her bathrobe. "Go back to sleep."

Rozanne grabbed her mother's hand and they walked down the hall to her bedroom. After her mother had tucked her back into bed she said, "Now, now. Tell me what's scaring you so much?"

Rozanne pointed to the window next to her bed. "It's the rain, Mama. Can't you hear it? It's coming down so hard on the porch roof. It woke me up and I felt afraid."

Mother looked at the window, listened and understood. The fiberglass roof magnified the sound that the falling water made. She reached over and stroked her little girl's blond curls. "Rozanne, rain is nothing to feel afraid of, don't you know that? Rain is good."

"Why?" Rozanne asked.

Mother smiled. "Because it helps the farmer grow crops so that we have food to eat. It gives us water to drink. It waters our lawns and flowers so they are beautiful."

Rozanne snuggled under the covers. "But it sounds so scary when it hits the roof."

Mother nodded in agreement. "It does, doesn't it?" Thinking quickly she added, "Here's something you don't know…Some people say that when it's raining, heaven is crying."

"Heaven crying?" the little girl said, amazed at the thought. "What does that mean?"

"Rozanne, do you remember Noah and the Ark?" asked Mother.

"Oh, yes! You read me the book about it and my primary teacher told us the story, too. It's neat—all about the animals and everything." Rozanne stopped talking and frowned. "But people drowned in the water, didn't they? That isn't nice—that's scary!"

"Let me tell you about that," Mother responded. "There once was a very righteous prophet named Enoch. He was probably one of the best men who ever lived on the earth. In fact, he was so good that he taught a lot of people about Heavenly Father and they became very righteous, as well. They all became so righteous that Heavenly Father took a whole city up into Heaven to be with him."

Rozanne's eyes widened as she imagined the scene. "I wish I could have seen it! That would be neat to see all of the people and the buildings and everything go up into heaven!"

Mother laughed. "Yes, that would be wonderful, wouldn't it? But before that happened, the Lord showed Enoch all of his creations and what was going to happen to them. The people that were left on the earth were very wicked. In fact, the Lord told Enoch that these wicked people would be the very people who would be drowned by the big flood."

"Really?" Rozanne wondered.

"Really," her mother replied before continuing the story. "When the Lord was showing these things to Enoch he started to cry."

Rozanne looked at her mother incredulously. She couldn't imagine such a thing. "The Lord cried?" she questioned.

Mother nodded. "Yes, he cried and Enoch was so surprised to see it. He asked the Lord why he was crying. The Lord told him he was crying because these people, who were so wicked, were still his children and he loved them. He felt so unhappy that they were doing such terrible things that he cried for them. He wants his us to be happy. We can't be happy when we are wicked, but even if we are, the Lord still loves us. You are his child and he loves you, no matter what. Don't ever forget that, Rozanne. Don't ever forget that."

Rozanne walked slowly down the hall after leaving Macie. Macie was one of the most confusing people she had ever met. She couldn't imagine Macie on a mission. She must have been very different when she left for the mission field.

"What's wrong?" said a voice to her left. She looked up to see Dr. Beall standing in the doorway of the room they used for her sessions.

"I've been talking to one of the patients here," she answered. "She's having a lot of problems. She wanted to talk to me, so I tried to help her. I don't know if I was able to help."

"I understand," Dr. Beall nodded. "It is time for your session now," he said, pointing to their accustomed room. "Do you want to come in and get started?"

"All right," she said as entered the room. "What do you want to talk about today."

Dr. Beall reached into his briefcase and pulled out her folder. After he had flipped through his notes he stated, "I want to talk some more about the school where you are teaching. Tell me more about it."

The topic surprised Rozanne. She thought they had already gone over it. "Like what?" she asked.

Dr. Beall took a yellow legal pad from the briefcase. "How many students did you say you have?"

She shrugged her shoulders. "Let me see...I figured it out the other day..." Quickly she added the enrollment of the six classes. "About two hundred and thirty-eight," she responded. "Why?"

Dr. Beall scowled slightly and wrote something on the pad. "I think I already told you that that was too many. I never had even half that many in all of the years I taught school."

That was disconcerting to her. "Really?"

Dr. Beall finished the sentence he was writing and looked up at her. "Rozanne, I don't think you realize the situation you are in." Tilting his head slightly he asked, "Do you want to go back to school?"

"I think so," she stammered. "I can't imagine anything else, but I feel sick when I think of doing it."

"I can't in good conscience allow that. I'm afraid that if I let you go back into that situation, we'll lose you this time. They are asking too much of you, do you understand that? Nobody—not even a music teacher—should have to take care of two hundred and thirty-eight students all by herself." He let that thought sink in before continuing, "How many hours a day would you say you worked?"

She shrugged apathetically, "At least ten to twelve. The other teachers all teased me about it. I got to know the janitorial staff quite well."

Dr. Beall's forehead furrowed. "I just simply can't allow that to continue. You have to get better. We have to get the situation changed or I won't release you to go back to the school. Do you understand what I am saying?"

"No," she answered, confused by what she thought she was hearing, "what do you mean, release me?"

Deliberately, he explained, "I am putting you on disability as of your admittance to the hospital. That means the school district will have to have me, as your doctor, release you to go back to work. I won't do that unless we can get some things changed for you. I prefer that you not go back at all."

"Not at all!" she cried.

"Not at all," he replied. "We'll explore other options and career choices before you make your final decision."

"But what if I want to go back?" she grieved.

"We'll just cross that bridge when we get to it," he replied. "I won't—I repeat—I won't let you go back into that same situation. It would be suicide. I haven't lost a patient to suicide yet and I don't want to start with you."

Dr. Beall closed the folder, put his pen into his pocket and the legal pad back into his briefcase. Folding his arms across his chest he studied her face. "Now," he began, "I want you to promise me something. Will you promise me that you won't hurt yourself?"

"Okay, I promise…"

"Rozanne, I'm serious," he insisted. "There is something about a patient promising that they won't hurt themselves that helps them not to do it. The climb back up won't be easy. I need you to promise me that you won't hurt yourself. I also want you to promise me that if you begin to feel unsafe, you will immediately call me. I don't care when it is or what time it is." He stopped and studied her face. "Do you promise?" he directed.

This time Rozanne waited before answering. She thought she could do what he wanted, but you never know what will happen next. She couldn't guarantee how she would react anymore. After considering the promises he wanted from her, she replied, "Okay. I promise you that I will call you if I feel unsafe."

Dr. Beall knew what she was leaving out. "And you won't hurt yourself?" he exhorted.

There was a long pause...

"You won't hurt yourself?" Dr. Beall asked again.

Rozanne still didn't answer him.

Dr. Beall sighed and crossed his legs. "Rozanne, do you have a plan for hurting yourself worked out?"

"...Yes, I do..."

There was a strained silence before he asked, "What is it?"

"...I don't think I want to tell you...."

Dr. Beall watched her. She was making a considerable effort to make herself melt into her chair. "Do you feel like hurting yourself now?" he inquired cautiously.

Rozanne shook her head.

"Then what's the problem?" he said, pursuing the promise he was after.

Rozanne struggled with herself. Why was she having such a hard time promising him not to hurt herself? She didn't want to do it—she knew that. It was too dangerous. It was too stupid. It would ruin everything. She could be lost forever...But still, she was having a hard time making herself make the promise. "I think that I just want to leave my options open," she said, trying to sound casual.

"What?!"

"No," she relented immediately. "I don't think I mean that...not really, Dr. Beall. Oh, all right," she sighed forlornly. "I promise...I won't hurt myself."

By the time she came out of the session with Dr. Beall, the other patients had left for lunch. Rozanne went to the staff window and knocked, "Hey, is anybody in there?"

She was surprised to see Clare. "I didn't know you were going to be here today."

What do you need?" he asked.

"I can't find anybody," she replied. Did the group leave for lunch already?"

Clare nodded. "Yes, quite a while ago. Where were you?"

"With Dr. Beall," she answered, watching him as he cleared off the desk.

"I see," he said. "Wait a minute. I'll get somebody to cover the window and I'll walk you down myself."

As she waited, she noticed Colby sitting in the group room all by himself. He was staring out the window. "That's odd," she thought. "Colby likes to eat so much that I can't imagine that he would choose to miss lunch."

When they got to the cafeteria and she had gone through the lunch line, Andy called out to her, "Hey, Rozanne! We missed you. Where have you been?"

"With Dr. Beall," she told him after she positioned herself across from him at the table.

"Hey, I've been wondering, "Andy said, "Did you ever call about the Workman's Compensation Insurance?"

Rozanne gasped, "No! I guess I forgot all about it."

"Why don't you do it when we get back to the wing?" Andy instructed.

"Okay…I guess I will…especially now," Rozanne replied. "Dr. Beall just told me he is putting me on disability from work. He blames my working conditions for my problem. He won't let me return to the school unless they are willing to change some things."

"It sounds like he'd back you on your claim," Andy said.

"Yes," she agreed. "I hadn't thought of that before. I believe you're right. I'll have to ask him about it. I guess you're right; I better call them when we get back from lunch."

As Rozanne finished eating her meal, she looked around the room. Laura and her husband were in the corner again. This time they weren't talking to each other. Laura was studying her food as she consumed it, as if she was afraid of what was on her plate. Her husband was looking around the room. He caught Rozanne's eye briefly before she quickly averted them. "How embarrassing!" Rozanne thought. "I guess I was staring at them. Laura's just such a mystery I can't help it."

She turned to Lizbeth and asked, "What's up with Colby? I saw him back on the wing. Why didn't he come down to lunch?"

"No one knows," Lizbeth said, bored. "He's not talking to us anymore."

Gloria added, "I think he is upset about something. Maybe the group this morning started to get to him."

"Colby!" laughed Lizbeth. "No way. I don't think anything gets to him."

"Still, something must be bugging him," said Andy thoughtfully. "Maybe something else has happened that we don't know about yet. I think we should just leave him alone for now."

"I think I may know what's wrong," Howard said. "I overheard him talking to his doctor. They are thinking about recommending to the court that he be sent to the penitentiary if he doesn't start working the program. He's probably pretty upset about it."

"That makes sense, doesn't it?" said Andy. "No wonder he's so mad."

"We better steer clear of him today," suggested Gloria.

Howard nodded. "Good idea, Gloria. Good idea."

Rozanne headed straight for the staff window when they returned to the wing and asked for her purse. She got the Workman's Compensation Insurance card out of its place in the plastic sleeve and went to the hall telephone and dialed the number. After a while a voice said, "Security Premium Care, This is Marlene. May I help you?"

"Yes. This is Rozanne Paxman. I teach school for Mt. Alta School District. I need to talk to someone about filing a Workman's Compensation claim."

"Mt. Alta School District?" Marlene repeated. "That would be Marsha's area. Just a minute, I'll connect you."

Soon Rozanne heard Marsha's voice say, "How can I help you?"

"I'm not sure," Rozanne began. "I think I need to file a Workman's Comp. claim."

"All right," Marsha said, "Why don't you tell me what happened?"

Rozanne told Marsha briefly what expired, what Dr. Beall was saying, and then waited for a response. "That's awful!" Marsha said. "I couldn't stand teaching middle school kids at all, let alone having fifty to sixty kids in a room! No wonder you had problems. It sounds like it is probably a stress claim. I'm not sure about it yet, but I believe you probably have a case. You'll have to get a statement from your doctor saying that your breakdown is related to the stress at work. If you can, you'll probably be all right. I tell you what; I'll do some asking around and get back to you. All you have to do right now is file the claim."

"How do I do that?"

"Basically, all you have to do is to tell me that you want to file a claim." Marsha replied. "Is that what you want to do?"

Rozanne was surprised at the ease of filing the claim. She had imagined that it would be more complicated. "Yes…I think so…" she said hesitantly. "Yes, I want to file a claim."

"Okay," Marsha said. "I've got it all down. We'll let you know what to do next. At some point, your principal will be told what is going on. Is that going to be a problem?"

"I hadn't thought of that!" Rozanne said, feeling her stomach hit bottom. "I don't know how she'll take it, but I guess it has to be done. Go ahead and file the claim."

"Wow!" Rozanne thought after she had hung up the receiver, "Maybe I'm going to be all right after all. Maybe they will pay the bills for the doctors and hospital. That's all I want. I just don't want to get stuck with a bunch of big bills that I can't pay!"

That afternoon, Rozanne was surprised to see Rhaun running the Substance Abuse group instead of Carol. "Where's Carol?" she asked.

"She has a family wedding today. I'm helping her out this afternoon and she is going to take one of my groups next week," he replied, unnerved.

"So what are we going to talk about?" asked Gloria.

"Yeah, Rhaun. How are you going to make this group different? It's supposed to be a Substance Abuse group, you know." said Macie.

"I know that, but I thought I'd leave it up to you guys." replied Rhaun. "We had a major session this morning. Any ideas?"

"Yes, I have one," started Gloria. "I'd like to…" Gloria stopped mid-sentence and stared at the door with her mouth hanging wide open. Everyone else looked up to see what had caused her to stop talking.

It was Laura. Laura was coming into the room. Laura, who had never spoken to another patient, was walking across the room. Laura, who had never attended group, was sitting down on the floor in front of the long leather couch. Laura, who had acted like she was on a different planet than the rest of them, began to speak. "Hi," she said casually. "What's going on?"

Complete silence reigned as Laura fiddled with her pant leg.

"So," she tried again, looking at the floor, "what do you do in these groups? I'm curious."

Rhaun took the initiative. "We talk about issues and problems that the group members are having. Together we try to find some solutions. We were just deciding what we are going to talk about this afternoon. Do you have anything you'd like to discuss?"

Laura studied her shoes and then began retying them.

Rhaun decided that she wasn't going to reply, so he persevered, "Gloria, you were going to give us an idea."

"I do have something I'd like to talk about, if that's all right," said Laura.

"Sure," Rhaun replied, "it's all right with me. Does anybody have any objections?"

The room was deathly still.

"I have a problem," began Laura. "It's the reason I'm here. You'll probably be shocked by what I am going to tell you."

"Try us. You might be surprised," remarked Heather.

Laura looked up from her shoes at Heather. They studied each other for a minute and Heather smiled at Laura. Laura quickly looked back at her shoes. "I have two children. My son is three years old. He is delicious…" Laura smiled softly to herself, "He has thick honey-blond hair and green eyes. He's so smart. He's already beginning to read and can count to one hundred. I was very content just to be his mother…But my husband wanted to have another child—so we did. This time I had a little girl. I guess she's a pretty little girl. She looks more like my husband than my son does. She's six months old."

"So what's the problem?" demanded Macie.

Laura looked over at Rhaun.

Rhaun looked at Macie.

Macie looked at her pant legs and pulled a long thread out of the inseam.

Laura began again. "The problems began shortly after we came home from the hospital. My husband was so thrilled to have a daughter—too thrilled, I thought. He dotes on her. When he comes home he goes straight to her. He'll go to great lengths to find the baby, no matter where she is. Then he picks her up and starts to play with her and carry on about what a beautiful baby she is and so on. It just makes me sick…"

Laura stopped speaking. Several minutes slowly ticked by before Laura took up her narration again, "I know you are probably shocked to hear me say that, aren't you? I'm shocked to hear me say that. But the truth is—I hate my daughter."

"Hate your daughter?" cried Lizbeth. "You hate your daughter?"

Laura looked up at her. "I know...it sounds dreadful...even to me...especially to me. I don't know what's wrong with me. I think I must be a monster."

"When did you decide you hated your daughter?" asked Rhaun.

Laura looked from Lizbeth to Rhaun. When she saw that he was studying her, she looked back at her shoes. "It was when she was about three months old. I just kept getting more and more upset when my husband would pay so much attention to her. It began to feel like he didn't notice me anymore. I guess I started to get jealous."

"Did you think that he didn't love you anymore?" asked Andy.

Laura looked up at him. "Yes, I guess that was it. I began to feel like he didn't love me anymore."

"Do you think that that's true," he asked.

Laura looked back down and shook her head. "No, probably not. But I felt that way anyway. I still feel that way."

"I tried to get over it," Laura sighed. "I tried to tell myself that I was just imagining things and I tried to act happy, but as time went on it just got worse and worse and worse. Then one day, after he went to work, I decided that I had to get out of there. So I packed a bag for my son and myself. I took the baby over to my husband's mother. I told her I wanted to go shopping. And then I got in my car and I drove and drove."

"Where did you go?" asked Rozanne.

"Everywhere and nowhere..." said Laura. She hugged her legs tightly.

The group didn't know what to do. The patients all looked at Rhaun, hoping that he'd have the answer. Rhaun looked around the room at the patients before looking back at Laura. "Laura, are you all right?" he said.

"No," she whispered, "but I'll be okay in a minute." Laura hugged her knees tighter and they could see that her shoulders begin shaking as she held the sobs inside. At last, she took a big breath, wiped her eyes and looked up.

"I drove all the way to St. George," she continued. "I think I was going to go to California. Don't ask me why…I don't know anybody there. But when I got to St. George, I chickened out. I turned the car back around and drove back to my mother-in-law's house, picked up the baby and went home. I got home in time to make supper and my husband didn't know anything about what I did. I wanted to run away, but I realized that there wasn't any place far enough that I could run away from myself, so I came home. That night, after dinner, I told my husband what I'd done. He was so mad at me." Laura's eyes began to fill up with tears again and after a moment; they began spilling down her cheeks.

"What did you do?" asked Howard. "How did you get here?"

"The next day I went to my doctor. I told him everything. He told me that I probably had postpartum depression. He told me that it's not that unusual. He gave me some pills and told me that I'd get better if I took them. I didn't want to take them because I had been a drug-addict when I was a teenager. I was hospitalized twice before I finally licked it."

"Hey! You're more messed up than me!" hooted Macie.

"Shut up, Macie. Just shut up!" demanded Heather.

"Macie," threatened Rhaun.

Laura went on as if she hadn't heard anyone, "I probably should have taken the medicine."

"What makes you say that?" asked Andy.

Laura glared at Andy. "I should have taken the medicine," she replied intensely, "because then I wouldn't have gotten so depressed. I should have taken it, but I was too scared…scared that I'd get addicted again. I'm still too scared to take it. Crazy, huh?"

Andy shook his head at her in reply.

Laura looked away from his kind gaze. "Anyway," she continued. "I got so depressed that I locked myself in the bathroom one night, about midnight, and swallowed the whole thing…the whole bottle of pills and whatever else I managed to dig up in our medicine cabinet. You know, like aspirin and stuff. I decided that I didn't want to live anymore."

The group gasped softly.

"I know...I shouldn't have done it," Laura said in response.

"What happened?" asked Heather.

"A while later, the baby began to cry. I didn't hear her, of course. I was out. But when my husband got up to take care of her, he couldn't find me, at first. Then he figured out that I was in the bathroom. He pounded on the door and yelled for me to open it up, but I couldn't hear him. He managed to get it open because it's the kind of door that can be unlocked by pushing a big nail in the little round hole on the outside of the doorknob. We learned that when my little boy accidentally locked himself inside once..."

Rozanne and Heather exchanged glances. They understood what Laura was talking about.

"Anyway," Laura continued, "he got in and found me passed out on the floor. He called 911 and they took me to the emergency room and pumped my stomach. I was still out of it. I guess they had a hard time reviving me, but they did. The doctors at the emergency room sent me here. After I got here my husband got me a different doctor. He's someone that doesn't usually deal with this hospital, but he has privileges here. Jace is a lawyer and has a lot of connections. Jace, that's my husband, got me a psychiatrist."

"What's his name?" asked Rhaun.

"Dr. Christofferson," replied Laura.

Rhaun smiled at her. "I know him. He's a good doctor."

Shrugging her shoulders, Laura replied, "Yes, I suppose he is. I've been working with him. I've been trying to decide what to do. My husband wants me to come home. I think I want to go somewhere else. I don't know that I should be around the baby."

"Why not?" Heather asked.

"I'm not sure what I'll do. But my husband says that I can't have my son if I don't come home. I'm just so mixed up about everything. I realize that

I'm not being rational, but I don't know how to turn myself around." Laura began to laugh nervously.

"Where would you go if you didn't go home?" asked Rhaun.

She stopped smiling. "I don't know…Maybe I'd go home to live with my parents for a while. But I don't want to be away from my son."

Rhaun looked at her intently. "Laura," he began, "has it occurred to you that if you begin taking your antidepressants and working with the doctors that you might begin working this all out in your mind. I think that the medications could help straighten out your physical imbalances so that the doctors could help you with your thought patterns through therapy."

"I know, I know," Laura said impatiently. "That's just what Dr. Christofferson tells me. He tells me that I'm not giving myself a chance by refusing to take the medications. I'm just so afraid of getting addicted."

"Laura!" Rhaun said, punctuating his thoughts with his moving hands, "Antidepressants aren't like that drugs you took when you were a teenager. They aren't addictive."

"That's what Dr. Christofferson says," Laura answered. "But how am I going to know that for sure?"

"Laura, you've got to try and trust somebody if you are ever to get well again," Rhaun replied. "You've got to try and help yourself."

"Ha! That's a laugh," she answered.

"What's wrong?" asked Rozanne.

Laura glared at her, irritated. "It's crazy to think that I could get well…that it will do any good to even try."

"I know how it is to feel hopeless, Laura," Rozanne stated. "That's how I felt before I came here. I thought everything was hopeless, but you know what? I don't anymore. I'm not saying that it will be easy. I don't think that at all, but now I think I can get better."

"Just how are you going to do that, huh? Just how?" demanded Laura.

Rozanne squirmed and looked around the room for help. The other patients were waiting for her answer, too. Rhaun was no help, either. He had a look on his face that indicated he was interested in what she would say. She knew that she had to try to put what she had been thinking about into words for Laura.

"I know that I am going to take my medications," she began. "Dr. Manning told me that it will take at least four to six weeks for them to start working, so I've got to take them for a while. I've got to believe that he knows what he is talking about. And I'm going to work at changing my thought processes. I'm going to write in my journal…I'm going to see Dr. Beall…I'm going to read my scriptures and pray…"

Laura pounced on that. "I don't even know if there is a God," she said caustically. "What's the use of praying if you don't know for sure there is a God?"

"I guess it's kind of like what you have to do to get well," Rozanne replied. "You have to hope that you will get well. When you are learning about God, you have to hope that he is there, at first. Then, after a while, when you act on that hope and pray and try to do the things you believe he'd want you to do, you begin to have experiences that tell you that he is there…that he loves you…that he is listening to your prayers."

Heather tapped Rozanne on the shoulders. "Do you really believe that?"

Rozanne turned in her chair and looked at Heather with all of the sincerity she could muster. "Yes, Heather, I do. I believe that God lives and that he loves us. I believe that he is concerned about us. I believe that he will help us. I have to believe it…I just have to…"

Dinner was over and Rozanne was lying on her bed, writing in her journal. Dr. Manning had just told her that she would be going home tomorrow and she wanted to sort out how she was feeling about this new development. She wrote. "I'm feeling very jittery and nervous tonight. Dr. Manning says its because I've gone through so many changes this week. This happens to me sometimes. I get this way and I have a hard time settling down and being by myself. Other times, I just want to be alone, almost desperately.

I'm nervous about going home because I'm cushioned here and cared for and I can talk about my thoughts and feelings freely with no one to tell me that I shouldn't feel that way. I don't have to worry about anyone else.

I have so many responsibilities at home. I'm going to have to make so many changes. I have to figure it out. I'm worried about becoming a couch potato again and about being isolated during the day. I'm not sure what Dr. Beall has in mind for me in therapy.

I'm worried about paying Dr. Beall. Can I get E.A.P. to finally refer me to him? Can the church or Workman's Compensation help pay my bill? I know that we won't have the ability to pay it. So many things are up in the air that it makes my head spin. I feel like I can't sort it out. I need to go home, but I'm scared to go home. I have to face it sometime…

I need to start taking walks—exercising. I need to learn to eat better. I need to find new outlets for my energy. I need to learn better ways of dealing with my children. I need to develop a healthier relationship with Gary. Maybe it is healthy, though. Even though he's carried me lately, in many ways, I've carried him throughout the years. Maybe that's what it's all about…being there to carry each other when times get tough.

I get the feeling I need to become more of a grownup, but is that just another one of those tapes in my head? Just because Mom always did everything for Dad, do I need to feel guilty about Gary helping me?

All of this is making my headache—I need to get some Tylenol.

She put the book down on the bed and rolled over and stared up at the ceiling. "Home…Why does that sound so intimidating?" she wondered, depressed.

"Rozanne, Rozanne…where are you?" called a voice.

"In here," she yelled.

Heather walked into the room. "Guess what? They're letting Laura go home! Can you believe it? She's about as messed up as anybody here. I don't think she's ready, do you?"

"No, I don't," answered Rozanne, shocked. "But the whole thing with Laura has been so strange, hasn't it? I don't understand her doctor at all."

Heather nodded her agreement before continuing, "There's something else. Gloria and Lizbeth are going home, too. This place is really going to empty out. But I saw an old guy with a beard checking in. He looks out of it. He's probably a drunk…"

"Probably," Rozanne said.

Heather sat down on the bed next to her and looked around the room. "You never know about this place. Sometimes it's completely full and other times it feels like a morgue. It is going to be so quiet tomorrow. It's Saturday tomorrow. On Saturdays we don't have any groups or anything much."

"Really?" Rozanne asked, "No groups? What will we do?"

Heather ran her fingers through her long, loose mane. "I just read and write in my journal. Some people watch a lot of TV. Nothing much happens on the weekends. The visiting hours are a lot longer, though."

Rozanne was suddenly relieved to be going home. It would be awful being here all weekend with nothing to do. The groups and sessions were helping her and it would be frightening not to have them. "I guess Rhaun and Carol need the weekends off," she thought. "I don't know why I didn't think of that before. Pretty stupid of me, really…"

"Rozanne…. Rozanne…" she heard as Rozanne felt Heather shake the bed to get her attention.

"What?" she blinked.

"I wanted to ask you something," she said, thoughtfully. "I've been thinking about it all day, but it has been on my mind a lot since the group meeting this afternoon."

"What is it?" Rozanne asked.

"You seem to sincerely believe in God," stated Heather.

"Yes, I do," Rozanne replied.

Heather pulled her loose, white sweater around her knees. "Do you know about him then?"

"I know some things about him," Rozanne answered. "I don't know everything, though."

"What do you think he would want me to do about my situation?"

Rozanne was puzzled. "What do you mean?" she asked.

"About being depressed…about the kids…about, you know, everything!"

Rozanne blew out a long breath. Why did everyone seem to think she had all of the answers? She didn't. She felt just as mixed up about everything as they were. She didn't know what to do about Heather. Heather's problems were worse than anyone she had ever known. "Please help me know what to say," she silently prayed.

She took courage and began, "I guess the first thing I need to do is to ask you a question."

"What question?" Heather replied.

"Do you believe in God?" Rozanne continued.

Heather contemplated Rozanne's question. "Yes, I think so."

Rozanne went on. "Then, if you believe in God, do you believe in Jesus Christ?"

"Yes, I believe I do"

"What do you know about him?" Rozanne asked.

Heather tried to recall what she had been told. "I know that he was born in Bethlehem. I know that he taught the people and performed a lot of miracles. I know that they killed him by hanging him on the cross. I know that he was resurrected."

"Do you know what that means?" asked Rozanne.

"What?" Heather asked, "to be resurrected, you mean?"

"Yes," Rozanne responded, "to be resurrected."

Heather thought for a minute. "I guess I've always thought that it means that he came back to life."

"Yes, he did come back to life..." Rozanne said, smiling, "but not to the same life he had before. He had finished his work. He had atoned for our sins so we could be forgiven. He was going to take his place at the side of his father, our father."

Heather nodded seriously. "You talked about us being forgiven. How does that happen?"

"We have to repent. We have to be baptized." Rozanne hesitated briefly before continuing. She wanted to be careful not to push Heather too hard. "Heather," she began again, "Macie told me you are a member of the Church of Jesus Christ of Latter-day Saints. Is that true?"

"Yes," Heather said, unfazed. "I was baptized when I was eight. Is has been years and years since I've gone, though. I probably didn't go long enough to learn much. So is that all, repent and be baptized?"

Rozanne sighed, "I wish...although, the repenting part is not so easy."

"What do you have to do to repent?"

Rozanne suddenly felt thankful for all of the Family Home Evening lessons she had given her children. "First you have to feel what the scriptures call a "godly sorrow" for your sins," she began. "That means that you have to feel sincerely bad that you did what was wrong...not just feel bad that you got caught."

"My kid's murderer doesn't feel that," Heather said angrily.

"I don't know..." Rozanne replied, "only the Lord knows what he is feeling for sure...but he probably doesn't or he would go to the police himself and confess."

Heather looked at her suspiciously. "What makes you say that?"

"If he felt godly sorrow for what he did," Rozanne answered hastily, "he'd feel so bad that he'd want to do anything he could to make it right. This leads us to the next step in repentance—you have to be willing to confess your sins. If they are small things, like personality quirks or things you should have done, but didn't—for example, you can just confess them to the Lord in your prayers. Although, I shouldn't make it seem so easy.

We tend to get quite prideful and have a hard time confessing to the Lord what we do wrong, even if the sins are small."

"What if they aren't small things?" Heather appealed.

"You have to go to the bishop or the authorities, if you have broken a law," Rozanne instructed, "and confess what you did wrong. If you have hurt someone else, you should also go to that person and confess to them, as well."

"That sounds hard," Heather replied.

"It is hard to confess what you've done wrong," Rozanne told her. "That's why it first takes a godly sorrow to be willing to do it. But it is such a relief once you have admitted what you did. It can feel like a big boulder has been lifted off of your back. It's quite hard to carry around a burden of guilt. Many people report that they feel so relieved that they don't care what happens next to them. They feel so much better that it's worth it."

Heather nodded. She understood now. "So then, once you've confessed what do you do next?"

"This is the hardest part." Rozanne told her. "You have to make it right. Sometimes…usually I think—it's not possible to make it entirely right again. Take your case, for instance. There is nothing that man could ever do to make it up to you. That's why sins like murder and rape are so serious. You can't make it up to someone. But if you can make it up, you should try."

Rozanne looked over at Heather to see how she was responding. Heather was intently considering everything she was hearing. Relaxing, Rozanne continued, "Then last and most importantly, you should change your life.

"Change your life?" Heather repeated.

"Yes, change your life," Rozanne repeated again, emphasizing the point. "You see, if you are truly sorry for something you did, you will do your best never to do it again. The scriptures teach that if you do it again after you have repented, the sin you have repented of comes right back on you. I think that when you are doing things that may seem common to do—like lying or saying bad things about another person—it is so tough! We have allowed ourselves to get into these bad habits and habits are hard to break. I'm having trouble with stuff like this…the bad habits, I mean. There has got to be something I'm missing…"

They sat on the bed in silence, each deep in thought. Finally Heather broke the silence, "You said that there was more than repenting and being baptized. What else could there be?"

"The Lord has said that we have to endure to the end," Rozanne replied.

"Endure," Heather sighed, "that's what life is…endurance."

Rozanne sighed also, exhausted. "Sometimes it is, isn't it? But I have a feeling that maybe it doesn't always have to feel that way. I hope that there is a way to be happy no matter what is happening to you. I've got to find the answer to this if I am going to enjoy my life again."

Heather wiped away the tear that had dropped onto her cheek. "Is that what the Lord means…that we just have to suffer through life? Is that what he means by endurance?"

"Probably a little," Rozanne answered. "He knows that this life is going to be hard for us. But I think that what he is mostly talking about by enduring to the end is to keep trying to do your best—to be good. Sometimes people are good for a long, long time and then they get tired and give up. If they would just keep going…That's one of the reasons I came here. I needed some help to learn how to keep going."

"Yes, I understand that," Heather murmured.

They sat in silence again. This time it was Rozanne that broke the quiet of the room. "Heather, there is something I haven't told you yet. It's something that I don't know if you want to hear."

Heather turned and met Rozanne's gaze with searching eyes. "What?"

"Are you sure you want to know?"

"Yes," Heather said. "I'd rather you tell me."

Rozanne painstakingly continued, "Do you remember the other day after you had hit the mattress? You turned to me and asked me why you didn't feel better?"

"…Yes, I remember."

Rozanne noted Heather's wary demeanor. She was afraid to say what she knew she had to tell Heather. Crossing her fingers for luck she made herself say, "I've been thinking a lot about that. I think that you need to try and forgive your kid's murderer."

"What?" Heather laughed bitterly. "Are you crazy? Forgive that no good louse?"

"I know…I know…" Rozanne said, trying to soothe her, "I understand, it must seem ridiculous to you. Certainly, it almost seems impossible. But that is what the Lord told us we have to do. He told us that we have to forgive in order to be forgiven."

Heather groaned, pained by the idea. "How can the Lord expect this of me? How can he expect me to forgive the murderer of my children? How can he expect me to do that?"

Rozanne searched her mind for the words to say that would help her understand. "Heather, if you stay angry at him for the rest of your life there isn't a soul on the earth that would blame you. It certainly would be understandable. But the Lord loves us and is merciful to us. He knows what is best for us and so he asks us to forgive."

"Why?" Heather demanded. "How could that be merciful?"

"Okay, okay," Rozanne said, putting her hands in front of her face. "I understand how you must be feeling to hear this. But just stop and think about this for a minute. Do you think that it's hurting that guy for a second that you hate him? Do you think it makes any difference to him at all? Do you think he even cares?"

"…No, probably not…"

"Probably not," Rozanne repeated to stress Heather's answer. "But now think Heather—think," Rozanne begged. "Who's hurting now? Who's suffering because of this hate? Who?"

Heather stared at the floor for a while. Then she threw her head back at stared at the ceiling until the tears began streaming down her face. Finally, she curled up in a ball on the bed. "Me. I'm the one who is suffering the most."

"That's right. Heather, the Lord wants us to forgive other people because he knows that it hurts us terribly when we don't forgive them. He wants us to trust him enough to believe that in the end the one who hurt us will be punished, if they haven't repented."

"It seems so hard," said Heather.

"You're probably right, Heather," Rozanne continued, "But maybe it would help to remember that the Lord loves you and he loves your children. He is just as angry as you are that your children were killed. He won't let that man get away with this terrible thing forever. You have to try and believe that."

"I think that I can believe that," sobbed Heather. "But it's quite another thing to forgive him for what he did, isn't it?"

"I know. It is," Rozanne said. "I don't even pretend that my situation is like yours, but we do have something in common. I have been carrying around some grudges for years. I realize that I have to finally get over it and forgive some people that hurt me a long, long time ago. It's hurting me—not them—that I am holding on to it. I am going to have Dr. Beall help me with it. I'm going to read my scriptures and try to find what I'm missing to be able to do it. I'm going to pray to Father in the name of Christ with all of my might for help. I know I've got to get over it for me to truly get well again. I have got to forgive them, so that I can get better. It won't make a bit of difference to them, but it will make a giant difference to me."

"He'll help us?" Heather said, sniffing quietly.

"Yes," Rozanne said, assuring herself as well as Heather. "The Book of Mormon teaches us that he never asks us to do anything unless he prepares a way for us to do it. He wouldn't expect you to do something big like this and then refuse to help you. He'll help you, if you ask him to."

Heather stood up and walked to the door without looking at Rozanne. She grabbed onto the doorjamb and said without turning back before disappearing down the hallway, "I just don't know...I just don't know...I'll have to think about all of this."

Rozanne sat on her bed, deep in thought for a very long time. At last she turned off her light and climbed into bed fully dressed. Right before she fell asleep she prayed, "Heavenly Father, in the name of thy Beloved Son, Please help us...Help us all..."

Day 5

▼

After breakfast, Mark told Rozanne she could get packed. He took her to the staff office and pulled her belongings out of one of the rooms she hadn't seen in the staff area. She shoved it all into the suitcase and carried it back to her room to finish the job. As she worked, she realized that this was one of the few times she had been alone in the past few days. Laura had gone home after Rozanne had gone to bed.

She stuffed all of her dirty clothes in the bag and then carefully slipped the pictures she had colored into the top pocket. She had finished eight of them. "I forgot how fun it is to color. I used to love it. I wonder what happened…I remember now. I gave it up because I couldn't satisfy myself. I convinced myself that if I couldn't do it as well as a professional I shouldn't do it at all. Stupid, stupid, stupid…"

Rozanne zipped up the pocket that held the pictures, closed the suitcase and then looked around the room. She didn't know what to do next. There was no group to go to…no schedule to keep…She felt lost.

After retrieving her scriptures and journal from her suitcase, she opened the book and began flipping aimlessly through the pages until she saw several passages of scripture that caught her eye, sending a cold chill down her back. They began with verse twenty of Alma chapter thirty-six, "And oh, what joy, and what marvelous light I did behold; yea, my soul was filled with joy as exceeding as was my pain! Yea, I say unto you, my son, that there could be nothing so exquisite and so bitter as were my pains. Yea, and again I say unto you, my son, that on the other hand, there can be nothing so exquisite and sweet as was my joy."

"Bitter pains…I know how that feels, don't I?" she thought. "But Alma said that his soul was filled with joy that was as great as the pains he had felt. He said that there is nothing that was as sweet as the joy he now felt. I can't imagine that. I just can't."

Tears began welling up in her eyes and soon her nose began to feel stuffy from the moisture. She had go into the bathroom to get a tissue. "I don't think I've ever felt that before…that kind of joy," she thought, as she blew her nose. "I think I've always been a little sad. But maybe not…it's so hard to tell right now. I do know that I've never felt the kind of joy Alma is talking about. I guess I've felt happiness before…like when my little children were born or when we adopted the boys. I know I was happy when Gary and I got married. I was happy in college…that was the best time of my life. But I don't think I've ever felt joy before."

The tears continued to stream down her face. She took a big breath and let it out slowly. "That's what I've got to find—joy. Oh Father in Heaven," she prayed, "in the name of thy son, Jesus Christ, I beg you: please, please, please…help me find the kind of joy that Alma talks about."

"Rozanne, your husband is here to take you home."

She opened her eyes, sat up and yawned. She had fallen asleep. "Okay, I'm coming," she answered. Picking up her books, she zipped them back in the suitcase and then carried the suitcase down the hall until she saw

Gary. He was smiling at her, "Hi, honey," he said as he kissed her on the cheek, "You ready to go?"

"I guess so," Rozanne awkwardly answered. She felt like bolting down the hall and climbing back into the bed she had just abandoned.

Mark interrupted their reunion. "Dr. Beall wants you to see him this week. He has already scheduled you for appointments on Tuesday and Wednesday at 11:00. Is that all right?"

"Sure."

Mark handed her some white slips of paper. "Here are some prescriptions Dr. Manning ordered for you. They ought to get you by for a while. You need to make an appointment to see him in two weeks. Here's his office number.

She took the papers from him and nodded. She would follow his instructions.

Mark reached out and shook her hand. "Good luck, Rozanne. Have a nice day at home."

"Thanks for everything, Mark," she smiled weakly.

Gary picked up her suitcase and they walked back down the hall towards the double doors that led to the outside world. Right before they reached them, Rozanne looked to her left and saw Heather's feet. She was lying on her bed. "Just a minute, Gary. There's someone I want to say goodbye to."

Rozanne entered Heather's room quietly. She had never been in it before. Heather had taped the pictures she had colored all over the wall next to her bed. Her nightstand was piled high with books. Rozanne could see that most of them were self-help books on various psychological topics. On the pinnacle of the stack was Heather's Book of Mormon.

"Heather, I wanted to say goodbye before I left."

Heather rolled over and blinked. Rozanne could tell that she had been crying. She also looked as if she hadn't been out of bed yet. "Are you going home?" Heather asked.

"Yes. Don't you remember? I told you last night that I would be going home today."

Heather wiped her eyes. "I forgot."

Rozanne's heart dropped to see Heather so upset. "Heather, what's wrong?"

Heather didn't answer. She turned her back to Rozanne and curled up into a ball. Rozanne watched her for a minute before saying, "Heather, are you safe?"

"Yes. I'm safe," Heather whispered.

Rozanne waited. She was afraid to continue because she had an uneasy feeling that she knew what was bothering Heather. She had to know for sure, so she asked, "Then what is it?"

"I've been thinking about what we talked about last night. I just don't know if I can do it."

"Do what?" Rozanne asked, already knowing the answer to her question.

There was no answer from the bed.

Rozanne just had to know for sure, so she tried again, "Heather, what can't you do?"

Heather moaned, "I don't know if I can forgive him."

"Heather," Rozanne said, "maybe you shouldn't worry about that yet. Maybe you should just try to find Christ first and then let him show you what to do about forgiving. Maybe forgiving that man is too much to start with…"

"Find Christ?"

"Yes," Rozanne affirmed. "You've asked me several times if I really believe in God…in Christ. I think that's the starting point. I mean, how can you forgive someone if you don't know forgiveness yet. Does that make any sense?"

"I guess so," Heather answered. "I'll think about that."

Rozanne sighed. "I've got to go. I wish I didn't have to leave you. You're the best thing I found here. Heather, I really care about you and what happens to you."

"Thanks," Rozanne heard.
"Goodbye, Heather…"
"Bye…"

Gary was waiting patiently for her when she returned to his side. He smiled the smile she loved the best. It was the smile he gave her when he wanted her to know that she was loved and protected. It was the smile he gave her when he wanted her to believe that things would somehow work out for them. It was the smile that never failed to make her realize that she was the luckiest woman on earth.

Taking his broad, warm hand, she took a deep breath and together they walked through the big double doors to go home.

Home

Journal Entry: November 2, 1996

    I'm home now. Gary thinks he has to watch the football game (typical). Andrew has a fever. Julianne's hair looks like it hasn't been combed in days. There are stacks of papers around the edges of dining room, even though I've asked Gary, repeatedly, not to sort papers in the front room. The neighbor just came over and informed us that not only has James and another boy been throwing rocks at their front door, they've done it before! Last time they made the boys paint their door. This is the first time I've heard about it.

    Gary went to get James. When they returned home, Gary was yelling at him to get outside and rake and bag up the leaves. James went downstairs and hurt Andrew and now Andrew is crying. I hear Gary saying, "Whose money did you take?" James yells back, "Nobody's!" Stephen yells something to James about his Sunday shirt. Gary goes down to talk to Andrew. James goes back out the front door. I look out of the window and can't see him. I'm a bundle of nerves. I've been home about twenty minutes. Welcome home, Mom!

Gary yells out the window at James, "Don't make a mess." My head is beginning to ache. I'm shutting down…What should I do about this? I can't solve everyone's problems and they don't listen to me, so I've quite talking to them. Help!

I've asked Gary two times to follow through with James about the leaves and he didn't. I reminded James that his Dad had told him to rake and bag the leaves. He said, "okay", but he hasn't started doing them.

I told James that I didn't want him to play with his friend for the rest of the day, because they've been in trouble. He promptly went downstairs and talked to Gary, who told James that he could play with Kyle. (He didn't think about checking with me first.) James is skillful at this "Mom against Dad" game he plays, and even though I've talked to Gary about it, nothing ever changes.)

I walked over to Smith's grocery store to pick up the prescriptions the doctor ordered for me. I also got some milk and a few videos. When I returned, Gary was gone and so was Stephen. After a while, I called Provo. Gary went down to his parents' house without telling me or leaving me a note on a day like today!

Peter from EAP called. I told him what happened to me this week. He agrees that I shouldn't be going to work, but he is still insisting that he could take care of this problem in two to four months at their clinic. That may be true, but now I am really attached to Dr. Beall. I just can't face changing doctors. I feel that Dr. Beall is my link to wellness. That probably doesn't make too much sense, but I feel like killing myself if I even think about the possibility of changing doctors. Peter says he'll talk to his supervisor and get back to me.

Why does everything have to be so rough? I feel depressed and panicky.

I want to watch "Big Business". It's a funny movie and I need something to get my mind off of all of this, but the little kids are watching "Toy Story". Oh well…

Journal Entry: November 3, 1996

I'm at church. I feel so sleepy and worn out…shaky inside…I've been playing the organ off and on for about twenty-six years and I did something today that I've never done before—I started playing the wrong song! Oops! During the sacrament song, the chorister was trying to lead the hymn faster than I was playing it. She wanted me to speed up, but I refused. I knew that I was going the right tempo—so I ignored her. I could tell she was bugged. I don't know how to take her. Her treatment of me so far has been designed to let me know that she wants to be in charge—kind of a mini power trip. I'm trying to ignore her. I don't have the energy to think about this annoyance. That's all it is—an annoyance. If she wants to make more of it then it's her problem. I sound like a brat, don't I?

Julianne is thrilled to have me home. She sticks to me like lint on wool pants. I wonder if I can learn to raise her in a way that assures that she has more confidence and people skills than I have.

I believe I used to be quite proud. Somehow, I grew up with the feeling that I was smarter, more special, and more righteous than other people were. I though that our family was better. I don't know where I got that. Nobody ever said it to me. Maybe it was just a self-protective response to the negative attention I received from the other kids. Who knows?

I have come to realize that this is not true at all. In fact, I have come to realize that I am a person with many problems and deficits. I have come to realize that even though I have a wonderful, very supportive family, they are just about as ordinary as they come. I have a deep desire to straighten myself up and become a better person without regaining the prideful self-image I use to own. I have been compelled to be humble. Now—Rozanne, learn the lesson well.

Later—

I'm home from church now. I can't believe what happened! Today is Fast Sunday, so we had a brief testimony meeting at the end of Relief Society. The Bishop slipped into the back of the room. I suspect he was there to keep an eye on me.

One of the sisters stood up to bear her testimony. She told us about her friend that had a nervous breakdown this last week and was hospitalized. (She doesn't know about me.) She said that she felt that her friend had a nervous breakdown because of a lack of understanding about Christ. She said that if her friend had a testimony of Christ, it wouldn't have happened. When she said that, the Relief Society President and the Bishop seemed alarmed. They both looked directly at me to see if I was upset by the remark.

There is just too much coincidence in the incident to blow it off. I've been going to church my whole life. I've never missed a Sunday unless I was too sick to go and I've never heard a testimony like it. You can't convince me that there wasn't something behind it. I don't blame the sister for saying what she did—she didn't know any better. In fact, most members don't know any better.

It's so sad. A lot of people think that if you're a strong member and try to be righteous, bad things won't happen to you. They think that you shouldn't get depressed, or have big financial problems, or have trouble with your children. I feel like there is a sensibility among some members that, somehow, the Lord will magically take all of your problems away and you'll live "happily ever after," if you try to be good and obedient. I think I used to believe that. I don't anymore. Bad things happen to good people…. (Who said that? I've heard that somewhere before…)

Journal Entry: November 4, 1996

I had a terrible time getting myself out of bed this morning. I got the kids off to school, then immediately climbed back under the covers and went back to sleep. When I finally got up, I watched TV before I was finally ready to ease myself out of the bedroom. I was afraid to start my day and my room was the safe spot. I was up and dressed by 11:30.

I raked the leaves a little.

I couldn't make myself eat, so I went to my brother's house for a while. My sister-in-law and I went walking. On the way home, I filled the van up with gas and I bought myself a McDonald's meal. I hid the wrappers in the trash so I wouldn't have to explain to the kids why I went to McDonald's without them. Then I watched some more TV.

It's hard to read. I got my new Good Housekeeping magazine and I just can't settle down to it.

Sent Stephen to the store for dog food.

Joyce B. called. She's in my ward and her daughter is in one of my classes at school. She wanted to tell me that she really likes me and to offer support. They are saying at the school that I'll be gone for two WEEKS! She telephoned here last week and Stephen told her that I was in the hospital, but didn't give her any more information. I couldn't tell if she was fishing for more information or what, but she did mention that I was at church yesterday. Now I feel very nervous and anxious…panicky…

I called Workman's Compensation today and it looks promising that I'll get 66 2/3% of my salary, plus my medical bills will be paid! I've got to talk to Dr. Beall about it. I've already called the hospital and told them.

I hid out in my room for the rest of the day. I'm not sure why.

I still haven't talked to mom—that's still ahead. I don't know when I'll be able to tell her about it. I'm not sure why I'm having such a hard time telling her. She'll probably be great about everything…she usually is. I'm probably being stupid again.

I just can't make myself cook, although I did do a little laundry and I picked up the upstairs.

One of my students called to tell me how much they miss me. I feel like I'm going to hyperventilate…

Later—

Didn't do too well after the phone call—I started having a panic attack.

Therapy Session: November 5, 1996

Rozanne sat in Dr. Beall's waiting room, her heart in her throat. The "needles-n-pins" sensation crawling up her torso told her that ever since she returned from the hospital, she had merely been surviving until the moment she could see him again.

She studied the small waiting area. Six chairs were placed around three walls and a small, child-sized table with chairs stood underneath one of the windows. Tossed across the table were several half-finished pictures and a couple of crayons.

On the right-hand side of the doorway stood a long, tall counter that held office supplies and a computer. Directly across from Rozanne hung "happy picture," designed to cheer up the unhappy people that came here, expecting deliverance from their sufferings. The corner, directly opposite the receptionist area, contained a small fish tank that housed twelve fish of various genus and colors, swimming around a rock castle and plastic greenery with obvious indifference to their surroundings.

Rozanne leaned over and looked through a pile of magazine on the table next to her in a vain effort to calm down, as she felt like a Chinese Acrobat Company was doing their routine inside her skull. Fortunately, it was only a few minutes before Dr. Beall came down the hall to collect her. "Hi, Rozanne," he said. "Why don't you come this way?" Temporarily relieved of the burden of her own thoughts, Rozanne gladly followed him down the short hall.

As she entered, she paused a moment to survey her surroundings. The room was the size of a track-house bedroom. That was good, she decided. It felt cozy.

Underneath a narrow, mini-blind covered window stood a long, tan leather couch with a blue, hand-crocheted afghan draped over one end. Rozanne hesitated. "Where shall I sit?" she thought, annoyed at herself for having trouble with even this insignificant decision. She chose the middle cushion. After she was settled, her eyes faced Dr. Beall's desk.

The wooden desk and matching hutch were made of dark maple. The shelves contained various books on psychological topics, pictures of Dr. Beall's wife and family, and the type of knick-knacks that are interesting to look at and hold. On the top shelf of the hutch stood a tall lamp-like object that had water in it with shiny colored metal pieces that shot up to the top and then floated back down. It was mesmerizing.

At the far end of the office, two large bookshelves were built into both sides of a window. They were crammed with books and momentos.

"How have you been doing?" Dr. Beall asked.

"Not too good."

Dr. Beall seated himself in the large, leather swivel chair at his desk. He frowned and looked inquisitively into her eyes. "What's been going on?"

"Here…Why don't you read this and you'll know," she said, passing her journal into his stretched out hand.

Dr. Beall buried himself in the book. "She really said that?"

"Said what?"

He looked up. "What the woman in Relief Society said about her friend. She thought her friend's nervous breakdown had been caused by a lack of understanding about Christ."

"Yes…she said it."

Dr. Beall grimaced and looked searchingly at her. "You don't believe it, do you?"

"No," Rozanne replied. "Don't worry. She didn't have the effect on me that she probably should have had. I'm messed up, but I do know that I have a testimony of Christ."

"Good," he nodded. "I thought you felt that way. It's just so odd. I can't believe you went to church at all. I didn't think you would."

"Why not?"

"It's not usual," he replied. "Most patients don't feel like going to church for a while after they come home from the hospital."

Rozanne clenched her fists until her knuckles turned white. "Dr. Beall, I had to go. I just had to. Can you understand that? I couldn't have stood the guilt if I didn't go. I know the church is true. I can't turn my back on that now, just because of this."

"I understand," Dr. Beall said. "Are you ready to begin? I'd like us to make a list of goals that we would like to accomplish during your therapy sessions."

"What kind of goals?"

"Here's an example," he answered. "You said that making the choice not to attend church would make you feel guilty. That may have been a perfectly appropriate response for the situation, but I have noticed that you tend to feel guilty about everything. Why don't we work on helping you to determine when you are experiencing appropriate guilt or inappropriate guilt?"

"I get it," Rozanne said. "I probably do need help with that. All right, that's fine. So what do we do now?"

"Open your journal and write down the list of goals we develop to work on while you're in therapy. I want this to be your list, though—not mine—so I'll expect your input."

"Dr. Beall, that's too hard. How am I supposed to know what to do?"

He smiled. "Just think about it for a while. I promise, it will come to you."

They sat it silence, Dr. Beall scribbling in his notes and Rozanne deliberately thinking about what he wanted from her. Finally, she told him she was ready. "I guess these are the things I'd like to work on: self-esteem…coping skills…guilt…different patterns of behavior. I'd also like to work with you and Gary to see if we can become more consistent with the kids. We need to be on the same page when we deal with them."

"I agree. I noticed that you are having problems with that when I read your journal. What else?"

Rozanne rubbed a finger along the leather piping on the edge of the couch cushion. It was smooth. It reminded her of a good leather purse, the kind that she'd never been able to own. "How about we do some more of that traumatic housecleaning that we did in the hospital?"

"All right," he said. "Anything else?"

"I need to start exercising, but I guess I have to do that myself, don't I?"

"That's an excellent idea," Dr. Beall said. "Did you know that when you exercise aerobically, your body releases chemicals that can actually decrease your depressive symptoms?"

Rozanne nodded. "I think I've heard that before. I guess I never thought that it applied to me, though. Silly, huh?"

"Not really," he replied. "Even though most people believe that exercise is important, they can easily come up with many pressing reasons not to exercise. It's hard to start an exercise program and maintain it." Dr. Beall placed her file back on his desk and sat back in his chair. "Now, I'd like you to do something that may be hard for you."

Rozanne pulled at a button on her shirtsleeve. It broke and she unsuccessfully tried to hold the two pieces together again. "What?"

"I want you to close your eyes and get a mental picture of something. Imagine you are with your mother. Can you do that? Good. Now, tell me—where is your mother's position in relationship to yours."

Rozanne thought about her mom. She was a beautiful woman. Rozanne had always been proud of her. "She's facing me."

"I thought so." Dr. Beall said.

"Is that important?"

"It could be," he answered. "Do you remember the list of tapes in your head you made while you were in the hospital? Let's look at that again. I want you to look at these items. How many of them come from your mom?"

Rozanne looked over the list. She felt embarrassed to look at them. "Almost all of them," she told him. "But, Dr. Beall, that doesn't seem so surprising to me. Isn't it our mothers who teach us almost all of our values?

These are all things I've either heard mom say or saw her do. She was such a wonderful mother to me that I guess I took all of these things quite seriously."

"All right. I can accept that. But let's look at the list objectively now. Are there any items that aren't absolutely true in every instance?"

"Actually," she said, hesitantly, "I can think up instances when most of them wouldn't be true. Some of them aren't true at all."

"That's right," Dr. Beall said. "Rozanne, I think that your relationship with your mother may need to change a little."

The thought made Rozanne's stomach clench. "What do you mean by that?"

"Think about your image of your mom and you together again. You said that she was facing you."

"So?"

"So…I think that it may mean that you still see your mother as your authority figure. Rozanne, how old are you?"

"Almost thirty-nine. I'll be thirty-nine on the eighteenth."

Dr. Beall pressed his fingers together. "Don't you think that thirty-nine years old may be just a little too old to still be considering your mother as your authority figure? Don't you think that it may be time to become your mother's friend, instead?"

Rozanne began to squirm. She didn't like where this discussion seemed to be heading. "I don't think I understand what you are saying?" she told him.

"You seem to treat your mother much as a very young child would. You look to her to help you make every decision. You look to her to validate everything you are doing. You almost seem fearful of making any decisions without her prior approval. Do you believe that this is true?"

Rozanne picked nervously at her pant leg. Was it really true?

"…Probably…" she answered.

Dr. Beall studied her face, watching her reactions carefully. "Rozanne, I'm not suggesting that you cut your mother out of your life. I'm suggesting that you move into a different manner of dealing with your mother. You need to treat her like a woman would treat her mother, not as a child would do. Are you beginning to understand me now?"

"…I think so…So what do I do about it?"

"To correct the situation you need to think of yourself by your mother's side," he replied. "You should be equals. Your opinions are just as valid as hers are. Your interests are just as valid as hers are. You should think of her as valuing you for who you are, not for who she would like you to become."

Rozanne felt her pulse quicken and her temple begin to throb. Even though she knew that he was probably right, she began feeling an enormous sense of disloyalty in this discussion. She began to feel guilty.

"Rozanne, you don't like this, do you?" he said.

"No, I don't."

"Why?"

"Guilty…just thinking about it makes me feel guilty."

"Why?"

"You should know. You told me you've been a bishop before."

"I have."

"So a bishop should know about honoring your parents and all of that."

"I'm not suggesting that you not honor your mother, Rozanne. I'm suggesting that you build a new relationship with her—a better relationship with her."

The breath that she had been holding squeezed out of her unbidden. She was annoyed. "Okay, I guess I can accept that. So how do I do it?"

"You have to take some time out and think about what you want out of the relationship. Then, you have to come together with your mother and try to make things different between you. You have to try to respond differently. You don't have to try to change your mother. You have to try to change how *you* interact with her.

It won't be easy for you or for her," he continued. "She won't know what's going on, at first. It might upset her. It will definitely upset you. But if you persist, in the end you will both enjoy the new, and better, relationship. In time, you may even be able to discuss the issue with her openly"

"It sounds hard," she said, pulling a face.

"It is hard. But I want you to think about this; you've told me that, sometimes, you feel that nothing you do is quite right. Is that how you feel?"

"Sometimes," she admitted.

"That's a symptom of an unequal relationship. You're old enough now, Rozanne. It's time to become friends with your mom. Now I'm going to make some statements that I want you to write down in your journal to consider. Are you ready?"

She nodded and wrote the following statements in her journal, feeling more anxious with each one:

1. The most important relationship in my life is with Gary—not my mother.
2. I must live my life. My mother must live hers.
3. My first responsibility is to follow my own heart and not someone else's.

"Okay," she said when he was finished, fidgeting nervously in her seat. "I'll think about them. Can we please go on to something else now?"

Dr. Beall leaned back in his swivel chair and crossed his arms behind his head. He could see she was unable to continue with this subject. "All right," he relented. "I'd like you to take the MMPI. It'll take a while, but it's not hard."

"What's that?"

"It's a clinical tool named The Minnesota Multi-phasic Personality Inventory, otherwise known as the MMPI. It's a method I use to help determine how you see yourself and how your relate to other people. It helps discover the level of depression you're experiencing and how anxious you are. It could be considered a snap-shot of your current emotional state."

"How do I take it?"

"It's not hard," he said. "It's very much like many of the computer-scored exams you must have taken throughout college—only this time you will be answering questions about how you feel and what you think. Do you think you could do that?"

"Sure," she replied. "It sounds easy enough. When I'm though with it, what happens?"

"I'll score it. Then we talk about what I discover tomorrow when you come. We'll use the scores to determine what areas we need to focus on in your treatment plan. Are you ready to begin?"

Journal Entry: November 5, 1996

Before I left my session with Dr. Beall today, he asked me if I have any hobbies. I told him that the only hobbies I had were taken away from me when I had my nervous breakdown. I used to enjoy music, but now I can't stand to think about it. My feelings about music are all mixed up with what happened to me at school. Music is the only hobby I've had for many, many years.

He asked me if there is anything I used to like to do as a child that I don't do anymore. It took awhile, but I finally remembered something; I liked to draw. I even took some art and painting classes in college. I gave it up because I felt that I wasn't good enough. If I couldn't do it as well as a professional, I thought that I shouldn't waste the time and money on it. "That's ridiculous!" he told me. "Go get yourselves some art supplies and start drawing again."

So I did.

What fun! I went to the local craft store and bought about $100 worth of supplies. I bought a portable art-board that has a smooth surface, a clip to hold the paper down, and an enormous rubber band that holds the paper still as you are working. I bought tons of professional-quality colored pencils. I like using colored pencils because they aren't messy. I don't feel ready to venture out into other mediums yet. I also bought drawing pencils, kneaded erasers, pads of art paper, and a metal pencil sharpener. I don't know what I'm going to do with them yet, but it will be exciting to find out.

Next, I went to the library and checked out a large stack of psychological self-help books. I believe that its time that I do something, myself, about getting better. Maybe I'll find something in them that will help me.

Dr. Beall also told me to start making lists of what I like and don't like. I told him that I tend to just go along with people, not expressing what I want to do, because I'm afraid that they will either reject me or make fun of me if they don't like my suggestions.

Okay—here goes…I like citrus flavors. I do not like butterscotch. I like to go to Friday's. I do not like to go to fried-chicken places. I like to watch ice-skating. I do not like to watch professional football….

Oh, this feels too, too stupid. I'll never tell anybody what I do or don't like, anyway. Besides, who cares what I like? Nobody!

I read something neat today. It was a statement by Helen Keller. She said, "Character cannot be developed in ease and quiet. Only through experiences of trial and suffering can the soul be strengthened, vision cleared, ambition inspired, and success achieved."

I like that. It gives me hope that maybe something good will come out of all of this pain I feel…

Therapy Session: November 6, 1997

Dr. Beall was leafing through a stack of papers as Rozanne entered the room. She sat in the middle of the leather couch, hearing the "whoosh" it made as she felt herself sinking into the softness. She took off her purse and placed it on her right side. That didn't feel right, so she moved it to her left side. The placement of the purse still bothered her, so she pulled her journal and pencil out of it and threw it on the floor. "What are you doing?" she asked him, trying to disperse the sense of awkwardness she was feeling.

"Looking at your MMPI scores. We have a few things to be concerned about, Rozanne." he replied, not lifting his head.

Rozanne opened the journal and began drawing tiny, tiny squares at the edge of one page. "Like what?" she asked.

"The report shows that you are still feeling dangerously suicidal. Is that true?"

She waited, hoping that she wouldn't have to answer the question.

"Let me read you this," he said, flipping to the correct page. "Most of the time I feel blue: true. These days I find it hard not to give up hope of amounting to something: true. I am happy most of the time: false. I certainly feel useless at times: true. I brood a great deal: true. Life is a strain for me much of the time: true. At times I think I am no good at all: true. The future seems hopeless to me: true. I often feel that I'm not as good as other people: true. I have recently considered killing myself: true. Lately I have thought a lot about killing myself: true."

Dr. Beall lowered the sheet and looked directly in her eyes. She looked away. "So it's true then?"

"…Yes…"

"Do you still have a plan?"

"…Yes…"

"Do you intend to use it?"

"…I…I…I don't think so…"

"Will you tell me what it is?"

She shook her head. No, she didn't want to do that. For reasons that she didn't understand, she didn't want to do that.

Dr. Beall tapped his fingers on his knee. "Will you promise me, at least, that you'll call me if you start to feel unsafe?"

"…Yes…I'm sure that I can do that, at least."

"Good. Let's go over these scores, then. Is that all right with you?"

Rozanne looked back up at him. His face looked weary. She gave him a small smile to indicate that she was all right, at least for the moment. He nodded and picked a stack of papers off of his desk and handed them to her. They were copies of her test scores.

As Rozanne studied the papers, she saw that several contained confusing looking charts. The remaining sheets were more helpful. Through them, she was able to tell that the basic idea of the test was to find out how she saw herself in various sub-topics of self-esteem.

She had rated high in only one area: competence. The test indicated that she felt capable of mastering new tasks, learning quickly and doing well at what she tried. Dr. Beall told her that that wasn't surprising, as she had proven her capability through achieving high grades in college and doing well as a teacher.

The test indicated that she saw herself as being average in her ability to influence others and being able to control herself. Rozanne agreed with that. She was probably no worse or no better than others in that regard. Next, Dr. Beall pointed out that she had low scores in five of the components of self-esteem, as well as in identity integration.

"What's that?" she asked.

"If you have a clear sense of identity, you know who you are," he told her. You know what you want out of life. You have goals. But the MMPI shows that you feel confused about what you want out of life. You also feel a great sense of conflict over who you are."

"I guess that's true…now…I don't think that used to be true," she said. "I think it got lost at Southland."

Dr. Beall nodded at her before continuing, "I'm concerned that you seem to feel unlovable, unlikable, and unattractive. We've got to work on this. You also seem extremely hard on yourself. Look at this," he said pointing to page thirteen. "You seem to think that you have some habits that are really harmful. What would they be?"

"I think you already know what they are, Dr. Beall. I check out of things. I isolate myself. I watch too much television."

"I don't agree with that assessment, Rozanne. Those behaviors may be a natural response to the stress you were under. They are symptoms of depression, not necessarily of a lack of moral responsibility."

She let his words sink in. She'd always believed that her symptoms showed a lack of moral backbone. Could it be true that these were just symptoms of a disease, like an excessive thirst, increased urination, weight loss, fatigue, nausea, and blurred vision were symptoms of diabetes? Could it really be true?

He sensed that she was have difficulty with this concept, so he asked her to look at page 12 of the report. "Let's go over the statements that indicate acute anxiety. Maybe it will help you understand," he told her.

Rozanne looked at the statements. They indicated that she feels unrested in the morning, unable to work, that she is under a great deal of tension, that her sleep is fitful and disturbed, that she has periods of great restlessness, that she feels nervous and anxious, and about to go to pieces. They also indicated that she saw herself as a high-strung person, with a sense that something dreadful was about to happen.

"Out of seventeen possible items in this section, Rozanne, you scored high on ten of them. These scores are indicative of acute anxiety. These are symptoms…symptoms. These are not indicators of someone who shows a lack of moral accountability. Do you understand now?"

"I guess so. It just gets so confusing to me, sometimes. There are so many things we are supposed to do as members of the church. I feel so guilty when I don't always behave the way I should. I thought I was just bad. I didn't realize I should be able to separate my symptoms from true sins. How am I supposed to know what behaviors are sinful and what behaviors are symptoms?"

Dr. Beall considered her question momentarily. How could he help her understand? Then he thought of something. "I think you need to start with the basics. Rozanne, what is the gospel of Jesus Christ?"

"The church."

"No, I didn't say the church—I said the gospel of Jesus Christ. Do you know what it is?"

"I thought I did, but now I'm wondering if I don't"

"I thought so. I'm going to give you a reading assignment. I don't usually do this with my patients, but I can see that your faith in the Lord is what is sustaining you. I want you to understand what his gospel truly is. I want you to write this down. Are you ready?"

Rozanne opened her journal to a new page.

"I want you to read third Nephi, chapters eleven, eighteen, and twenty-seven. I'd also like you to read second Nephi, chapter thirty-one. You study these chapters. They'll help you understand what Christ's gospel truly is. If you have a clear picture of these important truths, you'll find it easier to determine what is right and what is wrong. I think you'll discover that the gospel is far more simple that you've realized."

"All right," she said. "I'll read them."

"I'd also like you to read another book." Dr. Beall moved over to his bookshelf and pulled out a thick yellow paperback entitled, "Feeling Good—The New Mood Therapy," authored by Dr. David D. Burns."

"I already have that. I bought it years ago."

Dr. Beall looked surprised. "Have you read it?"

"No. I always meant to, but I guess I never got around to it."

"You start on this book. Dr. Burns teaches some excellent techniques for relieving depressive thought patterns and symptoms."

"Okay."

Dr. Beall looked at her, thought a moment and then said, "I'd like to do something totally different for the remainder of our session today. I'm going to teach you a method of deep relaxation I have developed by adapting various techniques. First, I'd like you to lie down on the couch. Take your shoes off, if you'd like. Cover yourself with the afghan and get comfortable."

Rozanne obeyed. She didn't remove her shoes, but she stretched out on the sofa and covered herself with the warm, royal blue afghan. She felt weird. "What now?"

"We have to pick a place that you find relaxing to imagine."

"Like what?"

"A lot of my patients pick the ocean. You're going to imagine that you're at the beach, enjoying the sounds of the waves."

Rozanne shuddered at the thought. "No! I can't do that. I've have too many dreams about drowning in the ocean!"

"Then think of a place that you do like."

Rozanne thought for a moment before she finally remembered one. In the mountains east of Cedar City, Utah, there is a lake called Navaho. It is a deep, calm, cold body of water, surrounded by tall, pine trees. She had been there several times with her parents and had happy memories of these experiences. "How about a mountain lake?" she said.

Dr. Beall nodded. That would work. "All right, then. Close your eyes and imagine that you are on a hillside looking down at the lake. It's a warm spring day and the air is still and peaceful. As you study your surroundings, you notice a set of large stone steps that descend down the hillside to the lake. As I count slowly to ten, you will see yourself walking down the steps. The further down the steps you go, the more relaxed you will feel. The further down the steps you go, the more peaceful you will feel. When you arrive at the bottom, you will feel totally relaxed, totally peaceful. Are you ready to walk down the stone steps?"

Rozanne nodded.

Dr. Beall began counting. "1…2…3…"

Rozanne felt her face and forehead relax.

"4…5…6…" his deep voice continued.

She felt her arm, leg and stomach muscles relax.

"7…8…9…"

She felt herself sinking into the comfortable leather lap she was on. She felt her eyelids grow so heavy that she imagined that she would be unable to open them, if she tried.

"10…Now you are totally relaxed. You don't have a care in the world. You look around and enjoy the beauty that surrounds the smooth, turquoise blue lake. You see the trees. You see the flowers. You see the grass that's growing next to the lake. Go over to the grass and sit down and enjoy the lovely scenery."

Rozanne saw herself walking over to the grass. She felt the cool blades of grass tickle her legs as she sat down. She saw the clear lake reflecting the majestic pines that surrounded the lake on three sides.

"Now…you look to your right and notice a country road that you haven't seen before. You stand up and start walking down the road. Soon, the path leads you over a small hill. It's a warm, sunny day and you enjoy the walk. When you come to the top of the hill, you see a vast expanse of rolling, grassy fields. A little way ahead of you, in a field, is a large, beautiful tree. You want to see the tree, so you begin walking down the simple, dirt road that leads to the tree."

Rozanne could see the tree. It was an enormous oak, with a thick broad trunk and expansive branches, making a large, cool shaded area under its canopy.

"As you approach the tree, you notice that someone is sitting on the other side of the enormous trunk. You walk around the tree to see who is there. Rozanne, who do you see?"

Rozanne looked…She was surprised to see a little blond-haired girl, her hair thick with should-length ringlets. She was wearing a sky blue dress and appeared to be about four years old.

"Rozanne, who do you see?" she heard again.

"Rosie. I see Rosie."

"Ah, Rosie," she heard Dr. Beall say. "Yes, it's Rosie. She smiles at you and reaches for your hand. What does she want from you?"

"She wants to sit on my lap. She wants me to love her."

"Then you must do this. Hold her in your arms and rock her. Sing to her. Play with her. Tell her stories. Show her that you love her."

Rozanne did as he said. She could see all of these things. After a while, Rozanne and Rosie simply sat there—enjoying the serenity of quite companionship.

Rozanne, now it's time to open your eyes."

Rozanne opened her eyes. She felt so calm and peaceful. She lay on the couch and blinked her eyes momentarily, before she pulled herself up to a sitting position again.

"Who's Rosie, Rozanne?" Dr. Beall said when she was upright.

"I guess that's me when I was a little girl."

"Why Rosie? Why not Rozanne." he asked.

"I think it's because I always wanted to be Rosie instead of Rozanne. My dad and Uncle Mont called me that, but mom didn't allow anyone else to. I had to be Rozanne. Rozanne was hard to spell. Rozanne was a name that no one ever got right. I wanted a nickname, but no one ever gave me one. I wanted to be Rosie, like my second cousin, Rosanne Hanks, got to be. Rosie seemed like a name people got who were loved. Rozanne seemed like a name that you got if you didn't have friends. Stupid, huh?"

"No, I don't think so. I'm going to call you Rosie now. How about that?"

Rozanne smiled, embarrassed. "Okay, I guess we can try it."

"Now, I have another assignment for you. I want you to be Rosie for a while. I want you to imagine the place where you went today. Go down the stone steps. Find the grass field. Play with Rosie and imagine that you are happy. Try to find out what Rosie would like. We know that she wants love. Every little girl wants love, but try to find out what else Rosie would like from you. Can you do that?"

"I'll try."

Journal Entry: November 6, 1996

Ugh! The more I'm reading, "Feeling Good," by Dr. Burns, the more anxious I feel. I can see myself in so much of it. Dr. Burns talks about distortions in thinking patterns such as "All or Nothing Thinking," (that's when you believe that if what you are doing is less than perfect, you are a failure), "Mental Filter" (that's picking out a single bad detail and thinking about it so much that everything starts to look bad to you), "Disqualifying the Positive" (that's when you believe that your positive experiences don't count, somehow), "Jumping to Conclusions", (through thinking you know what people are thinking or what is going to happen), "Should Statements" (trying to motivate yourself with "shoulds" and "shouldn'ts"…this makes you feel guilty!!!), and much, much more.

I didn't realize that my thought patterns have become so messed up. Maybe they've always been messed up. How did I get this way? How did I become so hard on myself? Guilt, guilt, and more guilt!

I'm starting to feel afraid to get well, even though I want to get well. Why is the thought of getting well causing me to experience so much anxiety?

I know. It's because if I get better, I'll have to take it all on again. I'm afraid I won't be able to cope and I'll eventually get worse. I can't imagine getting worse.

Later—

I've had a bad night—probably the worst night of my life. After I wrote that last piece, I began pacing around my room. My throat went dry and I felt so jittery. I suddenly couldn't stand the pain anymore.

I went back into the closet. Not the hall closet, like before, but the closet in my room. It felt safe to be in the dark, even though I had to sit on my shoes. I sat there, with the cool, silky feeling of my green Sunday dress falling across my face, wishing that I could slip down a rabbit hole into an alternate universe.

"If you want me, Father in Heaven, this would be a good time to come and get me," I thought. I wished desperately that it was my time to die, but there was no such luck. If I were going to die, it would have to be at my own hand.

I thought of my plan. I had a full bottle of Sinoquin. It's a liquid bottle of antidepressant that my family doctor in California gave me for my Fibromyalgia. Just the tiniest bit conks me out for the entire night, so I imagined that if I drank the entire bottle, I'd go to sleep and never wake up.

I sat in the closet and thought about the Sinoquin. I thought of going to sleep and never waking up. It started to sound logical to me. I thought, "I'm ruining everyone's life. I'm ruining the lives of my children. They would all be better off without me."

I sat in the closet, breathing the air that I had already breathed. It started to feel stifling, but I couldn't make myself leave the closet. I thought about the Sinoquin. I thought about my life. I thought about what it would mean if I took it. I thought, "Maybe Heavenly Father would forgive me. Maybe he'd understand how bad I feel. Maybe he'd understand that I'm in so much pain that I'd do almost anything to get the pain to stop."

I remembered that in my Patriarchal blessing, the Lord tells me that I need to be careful and that I need to remember that "through the actions of a thoughtless moment I could lose the blessings of eternity." I wondered if that meant that if I killed myself right now, I'd lose the blessings of eternity. I remembered that I knew the Lord was talking about suicide, even when I got my blessing at the age of fourteen. I never told anybody about that…. not even Mom…not even Gary.

I thought about what the blessing said and wondered if it was true. I was in pain. I was in terrible pain.

Emotional pain feels extremely physical. You can feel it in every pore of your body. You can feel with every breath you take. You imagine that you can even feel your brain hurting. You know that you feel your heart hurting. You want the pain to stop—to just go away.

"Heavenly Father, make it go away," I sobbed.

I waited.

I listened, but all I could hear was someone telling me that I was useless, I was worthless. They would be better off without me.

I crawled out of the closet. I crawled into the bathroom and struggled up the wall to get the Sinoquin out of the cupboard.

I held the bottle in my hand.

I looked at the bottle. Could I make myself do it? Could I make myself drink the liquid that would put me to sleep?

I stared at that bottle for a long, long time.

Finally, I made my decision. I wouldn't do it. I wouldn't drink that awful stuff.

At that moment—that very moment—Gary came into the bathroom and saw me. He grabbed the bottle and emptied it into the toilet and flushed it away.

I began to sob. I was glad that he had done it for me.

He carried me to bed and called Dr. Beall. I'm going to see him again tomorrow.

I made it. I'm still alive.

Therapy Session: November 7, 1996

"So, do you want to tell me about last night?"

Rozanne looked up from the black concentric circles she was vigorously scribbling in her journal. "I'm not sure."

"What happened?"

"I got afraid."

"Afraid of what?"

Rozanne continued scrawling the dark, ugly spirals that bumped angrily on top of each other on the page. She was really mad at herself. She was a loser.

"Afraid of what?" Dr. Beall repeated.

Rozanne's pen stopped moving. "Afraid of getting better."

"I see. Why does the thought of getting better feel so threatening to you?"

"I'm not sure it threatens me."

"Of course it does. You almost took your life last night because you felt so threatened. Now, are you going to tell me or not?"

Rozanne began scribbling spirals again. "Okay, I'll tell you." She continued moving her pen until she discovered that she was wearing a hole in the page.

She sighed and looked at the colored metal fragments doing their dance in the water of the tall lamp on Dr. Beall's desktop. The particles floated slowly down until they came in contact with an internal jet of water. The force of this stream propelled them up to the surface where they began floating dizzily down again.

"Rosie?" she heard.

Rozanne grimaced. "Right now—while I'm too sick—Gary is doing everything for me. If I get well, I'll have to start doing it all again. I'll have to work…and make sure we read the scriptures…and make sure we say family prayers…and make sure we have Family Home Evening…and make sure the kid's homework is done…and deal with the kid's teachers…and make sure the laundry is done…and make sure the groceries are bought and cooked…etc…etc…etc…I get depressed even thinking about it."

She stopped and rubbed vigorously at a smudge on her finger. "I feel guilty—so very, very guilty—that Gary is doing so much for me. I feel guilty when I think about the fact that Gary does all of these things for me and yet, I don't like some of the things he does."

"What kind of things?"

"Well, he isn't consistent with the kids. He threatens them with this and with that, but he never follows through. They know they can get away with everything, when he's around, and they do. When I'm alone with them, I can make them do things. But when he's there, no one listens to me. I feel guilty and disloyal even telling you that, Dr. Beall."

Dr. Beall considered what she was telling him. "How about we have your family come in for a meeting with me? Maybe I could help you with this. Do you want to try?"

"Okay."

"Rosie, now I want to have you do something. I am going to start a sentence and you give me an ending for it. This is the sentence: I am scared because…"

Rozanne considered her answer. What was she afraid of? "I have to make choices," she said, at last.

"I am scared because…" Dr. Beall's voice continued evenly.

"I'll probably fail."

"I'm scared because…"

"I don't know if I can do it."

"I am scared because…"

"I don't know what to do about the kids."

"I am scared because…"

"It's hard to live up to other people's expectations."

"I am scared because…"

"I might make our situation worse than it already is."

"I am scared because…"

"What if I regret giving up teaching?"

"I am scared because…"

"I'm flaky."

"I am scared because…"

"I don't know what I like to do."

"I am scared because…"

"I let other people tell me what to do…"

"I am scared because…"

"I'm having a hard time figuring it all out. What if Gary gets tired of waiting for me?"

Rozanne put her head in her hands and moaned. "That's enough, Dr. Beall. That's enough."

"All right. Why don't we visit Rosie now?"

Rozanne lay down on the couch in relief. She was exhausted and as she heard Dr. Beall's deep, soothing voice count to ten, it was no trouble to imagine herself by the side of the beautiful lake.

"I want you go walk over the hill now. Can you see Rosie?"

"Yes. She's waving at me."

"Go to her and take her in your arms. See what she wants to tell you today."

Rozanne felt Rosie's soft, chubby cheeks against hers as she lifted the little girl in her arms. She sat under the tree and asked Rosie to tell her what she wanted Rozanne to know.

"She's crying, Dr. Beall. She's crying."

"Why is she crying?"

"She says that her Grandma doesn't love her as much as she loves Rosie's cousins."

"Why does Rosie feel that way?"

"She doesn't know. She's just a little girl. She just wants Grandma to love her."

"Which Grandma is she talking about?"

"The one she looks like...the one she looks like."

"Rozanne, hold Rosie in you arms and tell her that you love her. Tell her that it will be all right. Wipe her tears and sing her a song. Tell her a story about a little girl who is loved. When you are ready, I want you to open your eyes."

Rozanne did as Dr. Beall's voice told her. She held Rosie and told her that she loved her. She sang a little song to her that she had always loved, "How Much is the Doggie in the Window?" That made Rosie laugh. She liked that song, too. When she was ready and Rosie seemed happier, Rozanne opened her eyes and sat up.

"Rosie, I want you to do something this weekend that will make Rosie feel happy," Dr. Beall said. "Try to remember what she always wanted, but never received, and give it to her."

"Like what?"

"Just listen to your heart. You'll know it when you find it."

Journal Entry: November 7, 1996

I had a rough day today. At Dr. Beall's office I remembered some tough things. The hardest was about my Grandma Warner. I'm sure she loved me. The adult Rozanne understands this, but I remembered how I felt as a child. I thought that she didn't like me very much. I always thought she preferred some of the other grandchildren more. I thought that they were welcome in her home and I wasn't.

I know now that she'd had some strokes that affected her ability to have her grandchildren around. I know now that she simply wasn't physically strong enough to deal with energy of small children. And I understand that I happened to be one of her youngest grandchildren. I was very little when she had her strokes and so I can't remember how she was before.

I can see how my own father changed when he had his stroke. He simply isn't the same person that he was before. He loves my children, but they wear him out. He's so weak. This new understanding has helped me to understand Grandma better.

She kept telling me how much I looked like her. She'd take out the pictures of herself as a young girl and say, "You look so much like me, Rozanne." But I didn't want to look like her because I thought that she didn't love me.

I do look like her. I have the same pale, white skin and the same round face. I have the same round figure, short hands and tiny feet. My mom and dad keep telling me that my personality is somewhat like hers, before she had her strokes. I don't know how I feel about that.

Oh, how I wish I knew her before she had her strokes. Maybe this ugly hole in my heart wouldn't be there. I wish that, somehow, she could let me know from the other side that she does love me. I wish…oh, how I wish this…

I used to console myself that—at least—my Grandma Stevens loved me. Now I know that I have just denied all of the pain and hurt I have buried deep inside of me all of these years. I feel it now and it's incredibly painful. My heart hurts.

Later—

I got out my art supplies and started drawing a picture.

"Pretty bird! Pretty bird!" chirped Topper, the blue parakeet, as Rozanne entered the pink kitchen. Rozanne crossed the room and stuck her finger through the bars of the chrome birdcage.

"You better be careful, Rozanne," said Grandma. "Topper just loves to bite little girl fingers."

Rozanne looked back at Grandma. She was wearing a yellow gauze dress with large, white daisies on it. Rozanne smiled. She liked how Grandma looked in that dress. It matched her pale, yellow hair.

"Would you like a bowl of ice cream, Rozanne?" Grandma asked.

"Oh, yes! Can I have pineapple on it?"

Grandma smiled at Rozanne. "Yes, I think that would be good. I like pineapple on my ice cream, too."

Rozanne climbed up on a kitchen chair. Her little legs dangled back and forth under the blue Formica tabletop. She saw Grandma come around the corner of the kitchen with the big, brown container that Rozanne knew had lots of vanilla ice cream in it. Grandma loved vanilla ice cream and always made sure to have enough to share with her grandchildren.

Grandma got a green bowl out of the cupboard and scooped a generous portion of ice cream in it before spooning some pineapple chunks on top. Then she placed the bowl in front of her eager granddaughter.

Rozanne put a big spoonful of the delicious mixture on her tongue. The slightly tart pineapple made an intoxicating contrast with the smooth, rich vanilla ice cream. "Mmmmm," she murmured happily.

"Pretty bird! Pretty bird!" chirped Topper. He wanted some ice cream, too. Grandma laughed. Rozanne laughed.

They were happy.

It made me feel better to draw the picture. I wish I could talk to Grandma. I wish I really knew who she was. I'll bet she did love me.

Journal Entry: November 9, 1996

I did something totally crazy today: I bought myself two porcelain dolls.

I decided to do what Dr. Beall told me to do. I went to the mall to see if I could find out what Rosie wanted. After I was there for a while, I realized that I'd always wanted a porcelain doll, but for some reason I didn't get one. It was probably because by the time I was old enough to take care of one, Mom had decided that I was too old for dolls.

I went to every store in the mall, looking for just the right one. In one store, I found a doll that I felt I needed to take home. She reminds me of how I feel. She has blond ringlets, blue eyes, wears a blue dress, and has an expression that indicates that she is on the verge of tears. I wanted to take her home right then, but I felt that if I bought her, I'd have to find another one to go with her.

I continued my search for several, exhausting hours before finding just the right doll. She, too, has blond ringlets and blue eyes, but she is wearing a pink-satin dress and a happy, peaceful expression. I immediately purchased her and dubbed her, "Rosie." Then, I went back to the first store and bought the sad doll, which I call, "Rozanne."

When I got home with the dolls, Julianne screamed with joy. She couldn't imagine that mom would buy herself some dolls and, of course, assumed that they were to be hers. She was disappointed when I took them in my bedroom and set them on top of my dresser. However, the disappointment was brief; she could look at them all she wanted to.

Gary looked at me like I was losing my mind, but didn't say anything. Later, he told me that I must be in my second childhood. I guess I am.

Journal Entry: November 10, 1996

I decided to do the scripture reading assignment that Dr. Beall gave me today. I drew a picture to help me understand what gospel of Jesus Christ really is. Here is one of the scriptures that I liked best: "Verily, verily, I saw unto you that this is my doctrine, and who buildeth upon this buildeth upon my rock, and the gates of hell shall not prevail against them." (3 Nephi 11:39)

I like that—particularly the part that tells us that if we build upon Christ the gates of hell shall not prevail. That's what feels like to be suicidal. You feel like you are facing the gates of hell, but you didn't do anything, necessarily, to get there. It's comforting to know that if I keep working on building my faith in Christ and following his gospel, that the gates of hell won't prevail. I can win! I can beat this!

I can see now that I have been making the gospel too complicated. The gospel isn't buildings or meetings or the callings you hold; those things are all just means to an end. It doesn't matter what other people think or say; what is important is my relationship is with Christ.

I guess that's what I need to do now. I need to stop worrying about everything and everybody else and just concentrate on Christ. If I do, everything else will naturally take care of itself.

Therapy Session: November 12, 1996

"Hi, Rosie," Dr. Beall said as she entered his office. "Did you have fun this weekend?"

Rosie. It felt strange to Rozanne to hear someone besides immediate family members call her that.

"Yes, I did," she said, "I have some things to show you." Rozanne opened the enormous shopping bag she had carried into the room and pulled out the pictures she had drawn, along with her new dolls.

Dr. Beall picked up the picture she had drawn of her Grandma Warner. "Did you realize that you drew her with her back towards you?" he asked.

That surprised Rozanne. She hadn't thought about it when she was drawing. "No, I didn't. I wonder why I did that."

Next, he looked at a brightly colored picture she had drawn and began to laugh. "Tell me about this one."

"That was a funny day. My brother, Mark, and I were helping Mom make some gingerbread cookies. Mom asked me to get the can of molasses out of the cupboard. It was on the top shelf and I was too short to reach it. I managed to grab the bottom of the can and the whole gallon of molasses spilled on top of my head."

"That must have felt awful!"

"It did! It was so thick and gooey. Mark has laughed about it for years. He loves to tell how funny I looked with the molasses running down my face and covering my glasses."

"How does that make you feel?"

"Oh, it doesn't bother me. It was too funny. I screamed and bawled and they laughed and laughed. I had to admit that it was funny. I drew this picture so that I could get in on the fun of seeing myself covered with a gallon can of molasses."

Rozanne picked out another picture. "Do you recognize this one?"

Dr. Beall smiled. "Yes, it's Rosie, isn't it? I can't believe what a good job you did. You're pretty good at this. You drew the field, the road and the tree just like I imagined them to be. I notice that you have drawn other scenes from the scenario, as well. Tell me, why did you do that?"

"I hang them on my bedroom wall. It makes me feel better to look at them. It also helps me to remember important things about myself."

"Tell me about the dolls."

"The one in the blue dress is Rozanne and the one in the pink dress is Rosie. I got them to remember that although I feel like Rozanne, I want to feel like Rosie does. I have one other thing to show you." Rozanne reached into the front pocket of her jeans and pulled out a polished piece of rose quartz.

"What's this about?" he said, reaching for the stone.

"It sounds silly, but I always wanted to have one. I was always afraid that everyone would laugh at me if I asked for a rock. When I was in the toy store the other day, I saw a box of them. I found one that fits the hollow of my hand perfectly. It feels smooth and cool. It only cost a dollar, but I like it so much that I keep it with me all of the time. Rub it and then put it next to your cheek. See? It gets warm. It picks up your body heat. I like to rub it and remember the rock that I am trying to build my life on."

"You've read the chapters I assigned you, haven't you?" Dr. Beall asked.

"Yes," she answered. "The quartz helps me to remember that it's the rock of Christ's gospel I should build my life on. If I get feeling upset, I rub it and pretty soon I begin to feel calm again."

Dr. Beall rubbed the rock. "I like that. You've done well this weekend." Then, as he handed the rock back to her, he asked, "Are you ready to talk to Rosie again?"

"Yes, I am."

As Dr. Beall told the story that led her down to the deep state of relaxation, Rozanne thought of the pictures she had drawn. She could see the gray rock stairs that descended the hillside. She could see the dark, cool, waveless lake. When she got to the bottom of the stairs, she imagined herself picking up a smooth, flat stone and skipping it across the glassy surface of the lake. It bounced a satisfactory six times before slipping under the water.

"Rozanne, I would like you to walk down the path that leads to the meadow. As you come to the crest of the hill, you see Rosie. She's waving at you. You wave back, but as you do, you're surprised to see that she has someone with her. You're curious about who is holding Rosie's hand, so you begin to walk to the tree. As you get closer to them, you are able to identify who is with Rosie. Who do you see?"

Rozanne looked at the two girls. At first, she was confused about who the second girl was, but then she recognized her and began to laugh out loud.

"What's so funny?"

Rozanne continued to laugh, unable to tell him.

"What?" Dr. Beall said, as he laughed at the sound of her delight.

Rozanne laughed even harder. Rosie and the girl were laughing, too. Rozanne was laughing because she realized that she knew this girl very well. This was someone she had totally forgotten about, but was overjoyed to remember. Finally, she was able stop laughing long enough to tell Dr. Beall about her discovery. "It's Ethel Pump!" she said, before bursting into laughter again.

"Ethel Pump?" he said, amused at the sound of the name. "Who on earth is Ethel Pump?"

"That was my nick-name in high school. It started when I went to music clinic one summer.

"Hey, Ethel!" Kim screamed with joy.

"Kim!"

The two girls rushed into each other's arms. It had been a whole year since the two had seen each other.

"What have you got planned, this year?" Kim smiled, her eyes twinkling.

"Oh, I've got a thing or two up my sleeves," Ethel laughed. "Just you wait!"

"Ethel?" asked a tall, dark, handsome boy who walked up behind Kim. "Who's Ethel?"

"That's Rozanne's nickname, John." Kim said. "Ethel, this is John. I go to high school with him in Mesa. He plays the trombone."

"Ethel? Why Ethel?" he laughed.

"Ethel Pump. You know—after the gasoline." Rozanne smiled back at him. He was cute. She wanted to get to know him better. "I got that name because I like to get things going."

It wasn't long before their laughter had attracted a large crowd of the many teenagers who had come from all over the western United States to participate in the two week music conference. Ethel was known to be a ringleader and she always seemed to have a big bunch of kids around her. But it was Kim, who Ethel wanted first and foremost, at her side. The two girls were becoming inseparable, as this was their third year together at the clinic.

The next day Ethel disclosed her plan. She had new clear, soft contact lenses. They were a new item and most people hadn't seen them yet. This is what gave her the idea. She knew that it would be impossible for an untrained eye to realize whether or not one was lying on the white, speckled marble floor of the Harris Fine Arts building.

After lunch they did it. Both of them, with a couple of close allies, got down on their knees and began looking for an imaginary "lost" contact. Of course, the contact was quite safe in Ethel's eye. But that was immaterial to their plan. They wanted to see what would happen.

It wasn't long before about twenty sympathetic individuals joined the search. Ethel remained cool. After a while, she looked over at Kim's profile to see her friend struggling not to laugh. Ethel decided that she better end the charade before someone guessed.

"Look everybody," she cried, holding an invisible contact high in the air. "I've found it!"

Quickly she pretended to pop it into her eye as the crowd clapped and cheered their relief. Ethel, Kim and co-conspirators shook hands and thanked all of the good Samaritans before walking calmly out the glass door. It was only *when they were safely around the corner they let their pent-up laughter loose in the hot, summer air.*

"That's the kind of thing Ethel Pump could do," Rozanne said, smiling at the memory. "Rozanne couldn't do things like that. Gradually, one or two of my close friends at home started calling me Ethel as well. It continued until I went away to college and Ethel was lost forever.

"She sounds like she was a lot of fun," Dr. Beall commented. "Why did you lose contact with her?"

"I don't know. I liked who I was when I was Ethel. I was relaxed and fun to be with. But serious old Rozanne kept taking over and Ethel lost the battle. Good heavens! I make it sound like I'm two different people, don't I? I'm not, but when people called me Ethel Pump, I felt different about myself and that was what made all the difference."

"Rosie," Dr. Beall said, "you can open your eyes now."

Rozanne obeyed, still smiling as she sat up.

Once she sitting again, Dr. Beall continued, "I'm giving you an assignment. I want you to be Ethel Pump all day today. I want you to do things that Ethel would want to do. I want you to think things Ethel would think. I want you to get in touch with the part of you that was Ethel Pump. Will you do it?"

Rozanne nodded. She felt excited even thinking about it.

Journal Entry: November 12, 1996

What a fun day! I had more fun that I can remember having in so many years, that I hate to admit to myself how long it has been.

When I left Dr. Beall's office I wasn't sure what I wanted to do, so I just started driving up 7th East towards downtown Salt Lake City. I began remembering all of the fun I had in Salt Lake when I went there on band trips with my friends. This gave me the idea that it would be a good idea to look around the city.

Suddenly, I knew what I really wanted to do; I wanted to go see the art exhibit in the Church History Museum. I just love to go to that museum, but whenever I've tried it before, I've had Gary and the kids with me. They aren't patient enough to let me stand and stare at a painting, just because I like it. It's always, "Come on, Mom. Hurry up, Mom. I'm bored, Mom. Can we go yet, Mom?"

I parked in the ZCMI Center parking lot and walked the short, pleasant distance to the sturdy, gray granite building that contains the three-story museum. There was a wonderful exhibit on display on the top floor. It had many paintings that were done by Latter-day Saint artists for an annual art contest.

One painting, in particular, moved me deeply. It was by Derek Hegsted and I believe he calls it, "I Will Not Fail Thee." It's a portrait of a young girl dressed in a flowing, white gown—she looks like she's about fifteen to me—and she is holding onto Christ's arm as she leans on the side of his bent leg. He's enfolding her in his right arm and stroking her hair with his left hand. The painting drew me in, as I imagined myself in the place of the girl, being comforted by my Savior. I must have stared at it for over a half-hour.

Finally, I had to know if I could own a copy of the painting. I impatiently rode the escalator down to the gift shop. Hurray! They were selling prints for ten dollars. When I came home, I immediately put it into a nice frame and hung it on my bedroom wall. (I'm developing quite a collection of things to display.) I love looking at the print of this magnificent work. It gives me hope.

After I had totally immersed myself in the wonders of the art museum, I walked around Temple Square, paying a long visit to the Christus (the enormous statue of Christ with out-stretched arms). Then I went over to Crossroads Mall and bought myself a yummy peanut-butter cookie that was dipped in dark chocolate. It was heaven.

On my way home, I went by the video store and rented several comedies that I particularly love and came home and watched them. Gary returned home from work during my feast of laughter and was surprised to see me in such a good mood. We watched the rest of the movies together and had a nice evening.

The best part of the day was how I felt as I imagined myself to be Ethel Pump again. I felt almost giddy with happiness. I found myself smiling broadly at complete strangers, my happiness amusing them so much that they soon were smiling back at me, despite themselves. I heard myself say a happy, "Hello" to almost everyone I met. It felt so good.

Why did I forget Ethel Pump? Why? She was so much fun. I've got to try to hang onto her.

Journal Entry: November 20, 1996

Yesterday I began a portrait of four "me's". That sounds eerie, I know, but let me explain…

The first "me" is Rosie. She's a little blond-haired girl that just wants to be loved. She is very simple and straightforward.

The second "me" is Ethel Pump. She's a high school girl that is full of life. She loves to laugh and have fun. She's outgoing and has the ability to draw people to her.

The third "me" is Rozanne. She's too serious. She's a good mom. She's a good daughter. She's a good wife. She's a good student. She's a good teacher. In fact, she's good at everything she does, but she is a very lonely, sad person. She's a stick-in-the-mud and has forgotten how to laugh.

The fourth "me" has an unknown identity. I don't know if she'll be called Rosie or Rozanne. She's who I'll become when I'm finally better.

I want her to keep the good parts of Rosie: the open and loving nature, the innocence. I also want her to keep the good parts of Rozanne: the accuracy, the thoroughness, the attention to detail, the desire to achieve and be righteous. I want her to definitely keep the fun of Ethel Pump. She needs to be able to laugh like Ethel can and to be able to see the fun side of life. I want her to dump the bad parts of Rozanne, though, like the insecurities, the selfishness, the pride, the too-serious nature, the sadness. I guess what I am saying is that I want to find all of the good parts of myself that I have lost, then keep and develop them.

I know that it might sound to someone who doesn't know me. They might think that I have multiple personalities, but I don't—I definitely don't. I simply have learned that we change as we move through the many different stages of our lives and as we change, we unwittingly become different people. Haven't we all met someone, that we knew a long time ago, that have become so changed through the passing of time, that we hardly recognized them?

Sometimes, we change in positive ways. Sometimes, however, we lose important parts of ourselves, like the parts that love fun, as the cares of life overwhelm us. I'm drawing the portrait of the four "me's" to hang on my wall. I'm a visual person and it helps me to look at them. It helps me remember that I intend to be a different—a better—person when this is all over.

Oh, Father in Heaven; help me to accomplish this most important goal. I ask this in the name of the Savior, Jesus Christ. Amen.

Journal Entry: November 21, 1996

I got up today and finished the portrait of the four "me's".

Bobbie, the secretary from Southland, brought a poster from my 1st period class. It had three candy bars on it and they all thirty-eight students signed it.

I got extremely panicky. I felt guilty. They want me to come back, but I'm not sure that I want to go back. It makes me feel like throwing up.

I studied six chapters in the Novell computer book that Gary has been encouraging me to read. (He thinks I ought to become a computer-networking engineer.)

I started two loads of laundry and put my rose quartz in my pocket.

Just thinking about the poster makes me feel dizzy. School just won't go away. It keeps rearing its head like an ugly pimple on my face.

I read a scripture in Romans chapter twelve that talks about everyone having different talents and how the Lord wants us to use them. It even mentions teaching! If I'm a good teacher, does that mean that the Lord wants me to go back to it?

Later—

I'm feeling confused. I think my head would float off, if it wasn't attached to my neck, I'm so dizzy. I'm out in my van in the parking lot of Dr. Beall's office waiting until my time to see him. I made myself stop thinking about what happened this morning until I got here, because I had a feeling this would happen.

I fall apart thinking about school. It was so hard. I felt so helpless...so abused. The kids were so mean to me. There is too much work to be done. I never could get caught up now, even if I worked twelve or fourteen hours a day, seven days a week. The more I do, the more everyone seems to expect from me.

Oh, help.... I'm drowning. Why can't I do something else?

Can I?

May I?

Why won't they just leave me alone?

Therapy Session: November 21, 1996

"What's wrong?" Dr. Beall said when he saw her face. She looked like a specter—a mere shadow of the person who he had last seen. "You better sit down." he instructed.

"Read this," she told him, handing him her journal, unable to say more.

Dr. Beall read the last entry in the journal and frowned. "What are we going to do about this?" he asked.

"You're asking me? You're asking *me?*"

"Not really, Rosie. That was a rhetorical question. I think that it's time for you to start exploring alternative career choices. We've put it off long enough, don't you think?"

"I guess so," Rozanne said, wiping her nose with the cuff of her sleeve.

Dr. Beall stood up and went to the bookcases at the end of the room. After looking through the stacks, he spotted what he was searching for. "I want you to read this book. Do the exercises. I've found that it's very helpful in situations like this."

Rozanne took the book from his hand. She recognized the title. She had seen "The Color of Your Parachute" in the library many times. "All right," she said. "I guess I'm ready to do it now."

"Good. Did you finish the assignment I gave you on Tuesday?"

"Yes." she sniffled, opening her Franklin Day Planner and handing it to him to read. Dr. Beall had given her the assignment of coming up with four principals she wanted to live by. She had finished them the day before.

"I'd like to copy these, if that's all right with you, and then we'll talk about them." When she had nodded her consent, he left the room.

"Loser…loser…loser…loser…" ran through her mind. "Those kids need you. You're selfish…loser…loser…loser…"

"Rosie, are you with me?" she heard.

"Oh…yes…I'm here."

"Let's go over your principals, okay?"

"Okay…" she said. Her mind kept running "Loser…selfish…jerk…. Loser…selfish…jerk…" over and over, like a bad marquee. She tried to listen to Dr. Beall. From a distance, she heard him read the list:

I take the time necessary to take care of my spiritual, emotional, and physical self.

I take the time to build good relationships with my husband and children.

I find the proper balance of meeting my family's spiritual, emotional, and temporal needs.

I find ways to serve the church and community in proper, reasonable ways that don't deplete my energy and distract me from what is truly important.

When he was finished reading, he reached over to the planner that was lying in her lap and circled three things on her list. The word "balance" from item number three and the words "deplete" and "truly important" from item number four. "Rosie, these are things that you need help with. I think that Gary needs to help you with these things. I would like you to bring your family in to see me next Tuesday, at 7:00. Will that work for you?"

"Sure," she said. She wondered if he knew how far away she was feeling.

"Open your journal. I have a few things I want to have you do as a family before then."

"Okay," she said, as she meekly obeyed. She tried to look attentive.

"Write this down: We will do these three things as a family before next week: 1. Family Prayer 2. Family Scripture Study 3. Family Home Evening." When she had finished writing, he continued, "Tell Gary that he's supposed to help you with this assignment. You're not supposed to do this on your own. He should help you, do you understand?"

"Yes." She doubted he would, but she would ask anyway. "Loser…Selfish…Jerk…" her mind screamed.

"I also want you to try and tape the children's interactions. You'll bring the tape the family meeting for Gary and the children to listen to on Tuesday. Can you do that?"

"I'll try…"

Dr. Beall sighed. He was trying to draw her into the discussion without success. He decided to change the subject. "End this sentence: I'm afraid to get better because…"

Silence.

"I'm afraid to get better because…"

Silence.

"I'm afraid to get better because…"

Rozanne wiped the tears that were running, unbidden, down her cheeks. She knew that her cheeks were probably covered with streaks of mascara. She knew that her nose was probably that annoying shade of red it always turned when she cried. She knew that if Dr. Beall could see her neck under her turtleneck sweater, he would see that her skin was blotchy. It always got that was when she got upset.

"I'm afraid to get better because…"

"…I'll have to do it all again…" she moaned.

"Rosie, I'm going to talk to Gary about this. You need him to be there with the kids. I mean, *actually* be there. You need his help disciplining them. You need his help taking care of them, don't you?"

Rozanne looked down at her lap.

"I promise you this, Rosie. I will try to get him to understand how important it is for him to take some of the burdens from your shoulders. If it's possible for him to hear it, he'll hear it from me."

Journal Entry: November 22, 1996

It's about 2:00 in the morning. I've been awake for hours. I can hear Gary snoring in the bedroom. The house is dark and quiet. The only light I can see is the dim reflection of the corner streetlight, filtering through the living-room mini-blinds, as it bounces off of the television screen. I've been curled up in the corner of the couch, drawing dark, ugly scenes of the fear I feel welling up inside me.

I had to draw. I had to let the pictures that were forming in my mind out onto paper. That's the only way I've found to stop them from haunting me. Once they're on paper, I no longer see them in my mind.

Now I only have seven hours before I see Dr. Beall again. I can make it. I can make it.…

I keep thinking about my students. I miss them. I love them. And yet, I fear them.

I wonder if I'll ever be the same again.

I used to walk into the classroom; secure in the knowledge that I would be able to be in total control of the situation at all times. Very little was able to get by me, because I seemed to have been born with an intuitive ability to manage a classroom. The best part of all was the love, the tremendous love I had for the kids. It made me happy just to be with them.

Now, everything has changed. I feel so cheated. I feel so betrayed. Why didn't the administration back me up? Isn't that their job? Why couldn't they see that they were losing a good teacher? Why don't they care? Why doesn't it matter that, with all of the teachers out there who are either apathetic or unable to really teach, the district is losing a teacher that put her whole heart and soul into her work? Why? I don't understand.

Unfortunately, I think the very qualities that made me a good teacher made me vulnerable to this situation. If I didn't care, it wouldn't have happened. If I didn't work hard, it wouldn't have happened. If I weren't concerned about the safety of my students, it wouldn't have happened.

Oh, sure...I've had some problems. But everyone has problems...Everyone...

Maybe if I had gone for help sooner. Maybe if I hadn't been so ashamed that I was feeling depressed and suicidal. Maybe I could have stopped it in time. Maybe...

But it feels like it's over now and I don't know what to do with myself. When I start thinking about what I'm going to do, I start becoming so afraid that I feel like disappearing. I feel like running away. I feel like going to sleep and never waking up.

I feel like everyone who ever made fun of me or laughed at me was right. I'm just a big joke. I'm the loser that they always thought I was. I'm just no good. They were right. I never should have thought that I could make it. See—how I feel now proves it. Everyone would be better off without me.

Gary would definitely be better off without me. Maybe he wouldn't have had so many hard times if he hadn't married me. Maybe he would have more money. I think that if I weren't here he'd be able to find a nice, normal wife.

The kids would be better off without me, too. See—I'm just messing up their lives. They're going to grow up and remember what I loony-tune they had for a mom. They're going to talk about it to everyone, and they'll be right. They need a mom who is strong. They need a mom who can lead them. They need a mom who isn't crying all of the time. They need a mom who can think about them and who doesn't get so lost in her own pain that they are pushed aside.

I can't stand it anymore. I can't *stand* it anymore. I just can't stand it…

Journal Entry: The morning of November 22, 1996—about 7:00

That was awful—so awful. But I made it, with Gary's help.

I went into the bathroom and found the enormous bottle of pain pills I had hidden behind the vaporizer in the bathroom cabinet. I sat down on the floor and held it in my hands. I didn't really want to die; I just wanted the pain to stop. I wanted the thoughts to stop, but I couldn't figure out how to make them go away.

I sat on the bathroom floor and sobbed. Gary woke up and found me. He took the bottle of pills away from me and flushed them down the toilet. I cried with relief as I saw them disappear down the funnel of water that took them out of my grasp forever. That bottle was the last part of my plan and now I'm relieved of worrying about whether or not to carry it out.

I wanted to get rid of them myself, but something was stopping me. I was glad Gary did it.

He took me in the bedroom and gave me another blessing. How grateful I am to be married to a worthy, priesthood holder who understands the power of a blessing. How grateful I am that he thinks of giving me a blessing when he sees that I need it.

He put his big, heavy hands on my head and told me that Heavenly Father loves me. Oh, how I needed to hear that. I began believing that Heavenly Father was so angry with me for the way I was feeling, that he couldn't love me anymore. He told me that everything would work out—that I would eventually be healed and that I would be happy once more.

Gary cast Satan out. When he did, I literally felt a darkness lift from me. It's hard to describe, but I felt him leave. I thought, "Why didn't I think of that? Why couldn't I have realized, myself, what was going on?"

When Satan left, I felt the Holy Ghost flood into my heart, filling it with peace. I was strengthened. I was able to sleep. I wish that I could understand how to have the Holy Ghost with me always. I need him. I know that now.

Therapy Session: November 22, 1996

"You had a very bad night," Dr. Beall said as he looked at the pictures she'd had drawn. "Are you sure you're all right now?"

"Yes. I had a blessing."

"Good. Why didn't you call me? You said you would call me."

Rozanne realized that she hadn't even thought of calling him, but she said, "It was the middle of the night, Dr. Beall. I don't think I could ever call someone in the middle of the night."

"Why not?"

"It's too rude. I think that I couldn't do it."

"Hmm," sighed Dr. Beall. "What would you like to do today?"

"I think I want to go see Rosie. I think she has something for me. I can't seem to go to her by myself at home. I've tried, but I can't do it alone."

"All right, then. Lay down and we'll go to work."

Rozanne snuggled under the afghan. It would be easy today. She felt so tired from last night's ordeal that she knew she would relax right away. She just hoped that she wouldn't fall asleep.

"1…2…3…" she heard Dr. Beall say, feeling the instant relaxation of her face.

"4…5…6…" she saw the pine trees that lined the gray-stoned path.

"7…8…9…" she could hear a bird screech, as it flew over the lake.

"10." She saw the patch of grass by the lake and started walking towards it. Something got in her way. She couldn't see what it was, but it wouldn't let her go to the patch of grass and sit down. "Can't…Can't…" she managed to say.

"Why can't you go to the grass, Rosie?"

"Someone is in my way. Someone is there."

"Who is it?"

Rozanne looked at the dark figure. She strained her eyes. The face was blurry.

"I can't see who it is."

"Try again. Make yourself see who it is," Dr. Beall instructed.

Rozanne squinted her eyes. The face slowly came into focus. It was Bailey—Bailey Rodgers! It was the same Bailey Rodgers that had teased and tormented her during junior high and high school. It was the same Bailey Rodgers that seemed to operate under the mandate that Rozanne's growing up years must be as miserable as possible.

"Bailey! It's Bailey. Why is she here?" Rozanne cried, squirming on the couch.

"Who's Bailey?"

"From junior high," Rozanne moaned.

Rozanne felt Dr. Beall place one hand on her head and one hand on her arm. "Bailey! You must leave Rozanne. You must leave her alone now. Do you understand me? It's time for you to go." He waited. "Rosie, has she gone?" he finally asked.

Rozanne writhed in agony. "Yes. She's gone, but now Jamie Kane is there. She's mad. Oh, she's so mad!"

"Jamie!" Dr. Beall ordered. "You go away. You've been in there long enough. I must insist that you leave Rozanne alone once and for all. Has she left, Rosie?"

"…Yes…but now Amy is there. She must have been standing behind Jamie. I don't understand why Amy is here. Why is she so mad at me?" Rozanne saw Amy's face laughing at her. Amy was always making fun of her.

Rozanne felt the hand on her head press down. "Amy! You've got to go, too. You simply cannot stay in there any longer. It has been long enough. Now…leave!" he dictated.

She saw Amy leave, but was dismayed to see someone standing behind her; it was Nicole—Nicole Kohlman. Nicole used to sit behind her in class and whisper—so very obviously—about what a jerk Rozanne was…how fat Rozanne was…how spoiled Rozanne was…

Rozanne's face twisted in pain. "Who do you see now, Rosie?" asked Dr. Beall.

"Nicole. Oh, it's Nicole. Make her go away. Make her go away," she cried.

The hand on her head pressed harder. "Nicole! You leave Rozanne alone. All of you—just go away and leave her alone. It's finally time for all of you to leave Rozanne in peace. Go, Nicole, go away. Never come back. You aren't welcome here anymore."

Rozanne felt her hands unclench. She felt the muscles in her legs go limp and she felt herself smiling. She liked whom she saw now. "Oh, look it's Martha! Oh, I'm so glad to see her. She was my best friend for so long…and now I see Valerie…I'm so glad to see Valerie. She was always my friend, no matter what."

"Rosie," said Dr. Beall, interrupting her happy memories. "It's time to open your eyes."

Rozanne reluctantly obeyed and sat back up on the couch.

"What was that all about, Rosie?" he asked.

"Those were the girls that used to tease me, Dr. Beall. I didn't know they were there. I can't believe that they were in there. I think that I've been letting what they said to me all those years ago roll around in my head. I think that I've been letting myself believe what they said when they were making fun of me. I guess I needed help getting rid of them, but I sure didn't know it until now!"

"Do you feel better?"

"Yes, I do. It's amazing. I feel I've been carrying around a backpack, heavy with steel plates, and someone finally took it off of me. I don't have to lift it anymore. What a relief! The best part is that suddenly, I don't feel mad at them anymore. I think I can finally forgive them for what they did to me."

Dr. Beall smiled, "Do you think you'll be all right until I see you again?"

"I do. I really do."

Journal Entry: November 26, 1996

We had our family meeting with Dr. Beall tonight.

The kids sat, lined up in a row from tall to short, on his big leather couch. Gary and I sat in chairs that Dr. Beall carried into the room. I watched my family closely for their reactions. I didn't know if they would accept what they were going to hear.

Dr. Beall tried to explain to them that I am very sick and that I need their help. He told them that if I don't get their help, he would make me live somewhere else, for a short time, while I am getting better. He told them that it makes it harder for me to get better when they are fighting and not helping each other. Then he asked them if they would all be willing to make some commitments to help me get better. They agreed and this is what the children promised to do: *Stephen:* 1. Clean his room 2. Inform me when he is going somewhere. 3. Do his chores. *James:* 1. Clean his room 2. When he comes home, he stays home 3. Stop teasing the other kids 4. Help when he's asked. *Andrew:* 1. Dust 2. Help when he's asked 3. When he is asked not to do something, he won't. If he does, he will be sent to his room. 4. Clean his room *Julianne:* 1. Stop screaming 2. Stop teasing brothers. 3. Do her chores.

They are supposed to report to Dr. Beall next Tuesday how well they are keeping their commitments. It will be interesting to see what happens. Gary promised to be more consistent. I guess time will tell...

Journal Entry: December 4, 1996

We had another family meeting with Dr. Beall last night and he got pretty disgusted with them. He made them report and grade themselves on how well they kept their commitments to over the past week. This is how they graded themselves: *Stephen:* 1. Failed 2. "D" 3. "I" *James:* 1. Good 2."F" 3. "F." *Andrew:* 1. 50% 2. "0" 3. Pretty good. *Julianne:* 1. "C" 2. "F." She stopped grading herself after numbers one and two.

Dr. Beall asked Gary what he had done to make sure that the kids were working on their commitments and Gary couldn't come up with anything to tell him.

I don't think I've ever seen Dr. Beall as upset as he became when he heard their reports. He told my family that they aren't doing what is necessary and that he may have to take me out of the home for a while so that I can get better. This agitated them all tremendously, but he showed no sympathy for them.

He looked over at me and saw that I was drawing myself up into a ball in my chair. He made them leave the room for a while, so we could talk privately. He told me that he wanted me to come up with a place that I could go, if it became necessary. He told me that he did not want to risk losing me to suicide. The whole experience really upset me a lot.

After the meeting was over, we took the kids over to the Arctic Circle restaurant that is across the street from Dr. Beall's office. We hadn't had any dinner and we were all feeling extremely cross.

I went to a table by a window and sat down, looking out at the street so that I wouldn't have to watch my family. I could see Gary's reflection in the window as he herded the kids to the counter and ordered some food for us. Then he brought my meal to me and we began eating.

The kids immediately began squabbling about nothing.

I couldn't stand to hear their angry voices, so I moved to a table away from them. I could see what was happening with my family, but I didn't want to participate in it.

Gary turned and looked at me as I ate. I could feel the tears running down my face. I could see them as they dripped off of the end of my nose. I could taste them as they fell on my French fries and made them soggy.

A look crossed Gary's face that I've never seen before. It was as if he woke up from a dream and was thrust into the uncomfortable awareness of how much I need him. He understood that I'm ill and that as his wife, I'm dependent on him for a certain type of aid that only he, as my husband can give. I need him to lead our family.

He snapped to attention and took charge of the situation. I heard his fierce whisper as he demanded that the fighting stop immediately. I saw the shocked looks on my children's faces as they realized that their father meant what he said, and their bodies stiffen as they realized that they must control themselves.

The children looked at each other in amazement at this development. They'd never heard their father speak in that manner before. They'd never felt, before this moment, that he truly meant what he said to them. There was a sensation among all six of us that things would never be the same again.

We ate the rest of the meal in silence. We drove home together in silence…and the deafening still continued to reign in our home as we entered it and everyone went to his or her room to ready themselves for bed. No voice was heard, except in whispers, as Gary gathered us together again for family prayer. Then—as we climbed in bed and the night covered us with darkness, lulling us to sleep—a tranquil hush covered us like a new, downy quilt.

Journal Entry: December 17, 1996

I have been looking for a job. Dr. Beall put me up to it so that I could finally decide whether or not I want to return to school. He calls it "exploring". That's what I feel like, too—an explorer. I'm in uncharted territory. I've never seriously considered doing anything besides teaching music, so it feels quite strange to think of myself in another type of situation.

Journal Entry: December 19, 1996

I have spent a lot of time at employment agencies and interviewing for jobs. It's a bad time of year to be looking for one, but I guess I'll do better in January when life gets back to normal after the holiday madness. I've taken typing tests, computer knowledge tests, grammar tests, and just about any other kind of test you can think of. It still feels so strange.

We are so broke, but we were blessed with help for Christmas. Gary's brother and sister got together and gave us some money. They told Gary that they knew what tough times are like and they wanted to make sure that the children had a nice Christmas. They are wonderful people. I just cried and cried when Gary told me about it. It made me feel so loved.

Journal Entry: December 24, 1996

I keep having dreams about my students. I keep feeling that I should go back to school. I feel guilty when I think about not going back. I know the kids miss me (well, most of them, anyway).

Today I told Dr. Beall that I'm thinking about going back to school. He turned red in the face. He tried to not let me know how much this upset him. He said, "All right, then. But if you're going back to school, some of the conditions you have been working under will need to be changed. What could the administration do to help you succeed, so that you can return to school safely?"

I gave him these conditions:

Someone to help out with data entry—this could be a student aide.

Either get someone else to teach the 5th period choir class or give me an accompanist so that I can watch the students at all times. I need to be able to know that they are safe in my room.

Give me the power to remove unruly and belligerent students from that class

Assure me that if I send a valid referral to the office about a severe incident, that the office will give an appropriate, serious consequence to the student(s) involved. I'm not asking the office to handle my duties in disciplining my students. I'm only asking that they back me up with consequences that I'm not able to give when the situation warrants it.

He wrote all of this down and then sat back in his chair in amazement. "That's all you want?" he asked.

"That's it."

He shook his head slowly, from side to side and said, "Rozanne, your demands are what any good administrator should give their teachers as a matter of policy. I'll be very surprised if you don't get what you want."

"Good," I said.

"Are you sure you want to do this?"

"Yes, I've got to try, Dr. Beall."

He told me that he would contact my principal right after Christmas vacation and talk to her about it. He'll try and work something out with her. I'll be on pins and needles waiting for her answer…

Journal Entry: January 7, 1997

Dr. Beall told me today that the principal and vice-principal wouldn't budge. They told him that they could make things better for next year, but that they won't change anything now. They wouldn't even consider getting me an accompanist for that one choir. He felt that the worst thing about the meeting was their absolute refusal to discuss backing me up when my students did something serious. He said it was incredible. He couldn't imagine an administrator reacting that way.

The worst thing that he told me was this: under the circumstances he won't sign my release to go back to school. He said that he's afraid that if I go back there now, without anything changed, he might lose me—once and for all. (That's a scary thought!) He told me that I came too close, this time, and he doesn't know if he could save me if I went back there, as things are.

So it's decided.

I can't go back to teaching school.

I feel like someone has died.

Journal Entry: January 15, 1997

I've begun working for First Security's Mutual Fund Department. Talk about a change! I don't think you could get any further away from teaching music, if you tried. I've been hired as an Administrative Assistant, but I think that my teaching background is part of the reason I was hired. There is some talk around the office of a future need for training employees. I think I'll probably be involved in it.

It's fun to get paid this much just to type and stuff things in envelopes. This is the kind of work I used to do as a teacher on my on own time. It's not very hard and I almost feel like I'm getting away with something.

I'm riding the bus downtown. It's quite an experience. It takes a long time to get there, so I have plenty of time to read the scriptures. I enjoy looking at the other commuters and listening to their conversations. I feel like I am in another world.

Journal Entry: February 10, 1997

One of the things I like best about my new job is my lunch hour. I get a whole hour. I never had that long as a teacher. I never had any free time to get my thoughts together.

Now that I have plenty of time, I walk over to Temple Square and look around. I love to go and sit in front of the Christus and think about Christ. I wonder what he thinks of me and my new life. I also love, love, love that I can go to the Church History Museum and look at the art exhibits anytime I want to.

Sometimes, I just walk up and down the streets of the downtown area. I've always wondered what it would be like to work down here. I imagined it would seem quite glamorous. It's not, but it is fun to see what is going on. There are many theatrical events, cultural events, and sporting events to attend. There is a constant hum of new construction. There are fun places to eat. I almost feel like I'm on a vacation.

Journal Entry: February 18, 1997

I've been learning about the Internet. I started by e-mailing all of the Paxman's I could find. It is an unusual name and we are all related, in one way or the other. I received e-mail from Paxman's all over the world.

After that, I decided to do something more constructive. I looked up all of my old friends' addresses. Over the years, I've gotten lost in the memories of the hurts I had received at the hands of some thoughtless kids. I had forgotten that I actually had a lot of friends. I especially wanted to contact the girls that were my age in my home ward and some of the special friends I had made at summer music clinics.

I was able to find them all! I had a lot of fun calling and surprising them. It was especially great to find one of my best friends, Kim, from Mesa, Arizona. We laughed and talked for a long time and promised not to ever lose contact with each other again. Why did I let my friends slip away through the years? Wouldn't Dr. Beall be surprised to know what I've been up to?

Journal Entry: February 26, 1997

I finally got the courage to tell mom what had happened to me. She was, naturally, hurt that I hadn't confided in her before now. She didn't have any idea that I wasn't teaching school anymore, although she did find it extremely curious that I didn't babble on about my Christmas concerts, the way I usually do. It was a hard conversation, but I think she understands.

She told me that she's had the uneasy sensation for months that something was desperately wrong with her family. She just didn't know what was wrong. It makes me feel bad to know this. I should have told her before.

It took me this long to realize, myself, why I didn't want to call her when it happened. It's hard to admit to your parents that you are a failure. It's even harder to admit to your parents that you can't handle life. I'm hoping that everything will be all right in time.

Journal Entry: March 24, 1997

We're moving! Life started to get too hard in Sandy. Too many memories...too many old students around and not enough friends in the area for our children...so we started looking for a new home. We were able to arrange to buy one in a quiet neighborhood in West Jordan. The house needs some work, but the area is nice and we have a good feeling about it. The payment is just slightly larger than our rent, so we'll be able to manage the finances well. I've decided that I am going to introduce myself as Rosie in my new ward. I want to try out the name and see if I like it.

Gary and I have enough money to go out for weekly dates and we are enjoying getting to know each other again. We are starting to get ahead, financially, a little now.

The bad news is that the District and their Workman's Compensation Insurance Company have decided that they don't want to pay for my medical bills. I contacted the state workman's compensation regulatory office and have been receiving advice from one of the men there. He has been very helpful. He told me that he thinks that I have a case, but that it will be precedent setting, if I win. That's why the district doesn't want to pay. They think that if they pay for my treatment, they'll have to pay for other teachers.

He referred me to a lawyer. The lawyer has accepted my case and in a few weeks I have to give a deposition. I have had to fill out tons of paperwork. I have also had to give them permission to send for all of the medical files for my whole life. I guess they want to see if I am, in actuality, just a crazy person. All of the doctors and the hospital are waiting to see what happens. So am I…I have to admit that just thinking about it makes me feel sick.

Journal Entry: April 8, 1997

I had a terrible experience today. I had to go to my family doctor to pick up a prescription refill. The route took me by the middle school I transferred away from to go to Southland. I left there to run away from the band teacher.

As I passed it, I was overcome with an enormous sense of grief. I felt like someone had died. I felt like my heart was being ripped right out of my chest. I thought to myself, "If I had just stuck it out there…I'm sure that things would have improved in time. But I *chose* to leave and now I've lost my career. Nothing will ever be the same again."

I pulled over to the side of the road and began to sob. I missed my students at that school. I missed the friends I had made in the building. I missed teaching. I thought that my heart was going to break.

I got home as quickly as I could and headed straight for my bedroom closet. I climbed inside and just wanted to die. I couldn't see a purpose for my life anymore. It wasn't until I drove past that school, for the first time, that I began to understand what I had lost. All I had ever wanted to be was a music teacher and now that's gone—snatched away from me in a nightmare.

I thought of all of the ways I could kill myself, but I didn't like any of the choices. Ultimately, I decided that killing myself wasn't an option at all.

I sat in the closet and cried for a long, long time. When I finally came out, I looked in the mirror. My tears had broken all of the tiny blood vessels around my eyes. I'm a mess...

Journal Entry: April 25, 1997

I just had the best time that I ever had in my entire life! I hosted a reunion for eight of my girlhood friends.

I'd already talked to most of them on the phone and one day I began thinking that if it was so much fun to talk to them on the telephone, imagine what fun we would have if we got together. I called one of the girls and asked her what she thought of the idea. She was just as enthusiastic about it as I was. We decided what we wanted to do, split up the list of women, and made the necessary phone calls to set the date.

We all made the decision that we wanted to have a slumber party, just like we used to do when we were kids. I sent Gary and the children down to spend the night with his folks and at 6:00 that evening, my friends started arriving.

After they were all here, I gave them T-shirts I had hand-painted for them. The shirts were yellow, with their names on the left sleeve. The front of the shirt said, "There's nothing like an old friend." We all put the shirts on and after we ate, we sat in a circle on my living room floor. We went around the circle and told each other what had happened to us in the past twenty years.

At first, we only told each other details that you would tell a stranger, but after time passed, we began to trust each other again and all kinds of personal things came tumbling out. It became as easy to talk to each other as it was when we were young. We realized that even though we hadn't seen each other in a long time, we still knew each other better than we knew other people. We stayed up almost all night talking.

It was a special experience, one that I will cherish all of the rest of my life.

Dr. Beall would laugh if he knew about it.

Journal Entry: May 2, 1997

I've been having a discontented feeling lately. I'm not sure why. On the surface, things seem quite good in my life.

I have a good job. In fact, the company is sending me to California this month to certify in a method of training employees. I think that I'll probably end up doing a lot of this in the future.

I have a nice home and the children seem to like it here in the neighborhood. They are doing much better in the schools in West Jordan than they did in Sandy.

I have a calling that I like. I am the Relief Society pianist. At first, I was called to play for the Primary, but it got so hard to be around the children and I began to feel so isolated that I got depressed again. No one talks to the Primary pianist. It wasn't a good situation for me at this particular time of life.

Gary decided to tell our new bishop about my nervous breakdown. He told him that he wanted me to get to know the other sisters in the ward.

The Bishop was understanding and told him that my name had just been submitted for the Relief Society job. I guess the Lord knows what I need.

I have a Visiting Teaching partner that I like a lot. She's the only woman that went out of her way to introduce herself to me when we were new in the ward. I was delighted when I was called to be her partner.

I also like the women we are visiting. One of them, Sarah, also struggles with depression. We hit it off right away. My partner, Mary, told me that other partners she has had in the past haven't been nearly as understanding of Sarah. They have had the opinion that she should just be able to "snap herself out of it."

I keep hearing this ridiculous idea. Don't people get it? Depression is an illness. It's not something you can just "snap yourself out of." It takes work—lots and lots of work—and medical attention…and prayers…and blessings…and love and patience from people around you. I sure wish I could tell people what it's really like to be depressed. Maybe, then, they'd understand and be more helpful.

Probably the top of my blessings I enjoy is the privilege I enjoy to have a husband who loves me and is patient with me. I have four wonderful children. I have parents and brothers who love me. I have in-laws who love me and treat me well.

Lest I forget, I have the true Gospel of Jesus Christ. That alone should be enough to make me contented.

So why don't I feel happy?

Journal Entry: May 18, 1997

I had a nice experience in California, although I missed the children while I was gone. It was a short, but extremely intense, course of study that taught us exactly how they want their materials taught to class participants. I had lots of homework each night and was relieved when the class had ended. I had arranged for Gary to fly in for the weekend and Saturday we drove over to San Francisco and saw the sights. It was fun to be with him, all by myself, for a while.

On the surface my life seems so good right now. I have few worries except the constant concern I feel for my children in the afternoons. They are on their own for about three hours. I worry about what might happen to them. But I'd have to admit that singular concern is not the cause of my discontent.

I still don't know what is wrong, but something is definitely wrong. The sensation of discontent looms over me like a hawk circling the desert, watching for an unsuspecting rabbit to appear out of its hole…

Therapy Session: June 5, 1997

Rozanne waited anxiously for Dr. Beall to appear down the hall and usher her into his inner sanctum. It had been nearly five months since she had last seen him and she was unhappy to be back. She felt like she had failed, as the need to see him again seemed to push her back into the dark crevice she had worked so hard to climb out of such a short time ago. She thought she had made it, but the very fact that she was sitting in his reception area told her that she had not.

At last she saw him striding purposely down the short hall towards her. He smiled expectantly at her, but her face felt frozen, unable to return even such a small gesture. "It's nice to see you again, Rosie," he said, thrusting his right hand towards her.

"I'm not sure I can return the thought, Dr. Beall," she replied, shaking his hand.

His eyebrows knit together as he frowned at her remark. "Shall we go to my office then?"

Rozanne warily followed him back down the hall and took her accustomed place on the couch after they reached his office. He was prepared for her. He opened his file and glanced at the last couple of pages of entries. "How's your job going? Do you still work for First Security?"

"Yes, I do. It's going very well. I have recently negotiated a pay raise and promotion. It takes effect next month—on my six month anniversary with the company."

"That soon? Tell me about it."

"I've been doing a lot of work on a training project for the Private Client Group. They are going to arrange specialists in five different states into teams. I will be flying all over the intermountain west, training these employees. This training project will begin for the largest group of employees the end of July. My new position, which is officially "Sales Training Coordinator," is a salaried position. My current position pays by the hour, so you can see it is a big leap forward."

"How do you feel about this change?"

"It sounds rather exciting to be flying around the western United States to all of those cities I've never seen before. I've always wondered what it would be like to have to travel with my job. I will be training employees in this area, as well. I've had to earn the trust of different people in the company to win this promotion. They didn't know what to think of me, at first. But my boss believed in me and slowly put me in situations that proved to them that I could handle the job. The progress has been slow—or at least it feels that way to me—but I believe that they're coming around. It's nothing like teaching middle school kids, though. I'm even going to be getting my own office."

"It's sounds like you've been successful."

Rozanne sighed. "I guess I have been."

Dr. Beall frowned and leaned back in his chair. "Why don't you tell me why you are here, Rosie."

Rozanne started to cry when she heard the question. The feelings of despair and depression that she had been holding in for weeks began to overflow the boundaries that she had forcefully set. She couldn't talk. She could only cry.

Dr. Beall handed her the box of tissues he always had handy on the top of his desk. She reached for it, took one out and blew her nose loudly into the white, scratchy surface. "Take your time," he said.

The comforting tone of his voice sent a fresh flood of tears coursing down her cheeks. Rozanne started to feel ridiculous. She didn't know why she felt so upset. "I don't...I can't.... Oh..." she sniffled.

"It's all right. We've got time. You'll tell me when you can."

"Oh, Dr. Beall, I don't know what's wrong with me now. I really don't. Everything seems to be so great. A lot of the problems I used to have are gone. I have a good job and I'm successful. Gary and I are getting along great and the kids are doing better than they ever have since we moved back to Utah. They seem very happy. They all have friends and are doing well in school."

"Okay, so everybody else seems happy. Tell me about you."

Rozanne began picking at the gold buttons on her suit coat. "I just feel lost. I keep finding myself feeling depressed and I don't even know why. One of the ladies I visit each month told me that she began feeling that way right before she remembered that she had been sexually abused. She thinks that's what's wrong with me. But I don't. I don't think that's it at all. My past feels cleaned up. I can't for the life of me figure out what's wrong with me."

Rozanne looked at the wall. "I just find myself feeling sad, and worthless...like my life isn't going anywhere...like I don't matter...It doesn't make any sense at all to me. I want this icky feeling to go away, but nothing that used to work helps me anymore. I thought I was over it. I thought I was well!"

"You're being too hard on yourself, Rosie. Did I ever tell you that it usually takes at least a year to get better, once you've had a nervous breakdown?"

"A whole year?" Rozanne cried as a rock hit the bottom of her stomach. This was distressing news. How could it possibly take a whole year to get better? She didn't think that she could even stand another week of this...

"Yes…a whole year…sometimes longer. But I think that the depression you are experiencing now is a different type of depression you had before. Rosie, can you remember when these feelings started?"

Rozanne made herself go back in time. Was it before she went to California? Yes…Was it before she had the reunion with her friends? Yes, it was. When was it? When was it?

Then she remembered.

It began the day that she cried hysterically in front of her old middle school—the one that she had transferred away from. That was the beginning of this new descent into this pit. It was a pit—a dark, dank pit.

The sad feelings had begun slowly, at first. Over time they grew, like ivy climbing up a wall, breaking down the surface of its host as it searches for crevices to cling to. She had become so depressed that each day turned into a marathon of fear, doubt, and hurt that she forced herself through, searching desperately for little moments of hope to cling to as she scaled her own wall of despair. At last, she had to admit to herself that she was over her head in the war she waged with this current bout with depression and she called the one person she hoped could rescue her—Dr. Beall.

"I remember now, Dr. Beall. One day, as I was driving to the doctor, I unexpectedly passed the first middle school I taught at in this valley. I looked over at that big, red brick building and it hit me: I will never teach school again. That life is over for me. I've lost my career. It's over. It's gone."

Dr. Beall nodded. "Rosie, I think I know what is wrong with you."

"You do?"

"Yes. You have what is called an "existential" depression."

"Existential?"

"Yes. Have you ever heard that term before?"

"I have. We studied it in several of my college courses. I particularly remember it in terms of a movement of art and music in this century. I remember the artwork being very dark, jagged. It came as an answer to the light, airy, almost transparent works of the Impressionist Era. My memory tells me that it came out of Germany."

"That's right," Dr. Beall said. "The Existentialist Movement was essentially a school of thought where people began looking for the meaning of life. The existentialists believed that human existence isn't necessarily describable or understandable in idealistic or scientific terms. Unlike prior generations, they began thinking that our existence on this planet may not be easily explained. That's why the music and art works were so different…angular…dark…filled with angst and discord."

"Okay…so what does that have to do with me, Dr. Beall?"

"It's pretty simple, really. When you were a teacher, you felt that your life had meaning. Now you don't. You've lost the meaning you attached to your life; that of being a teacher of young people."

Rozanne let this idea sink in briefly before responding. It sounded pretty reasonable. It was true that while she was successful at her new job, she found it less than satisfying, because the accumulation of wealth, for the simple sake of acquiring and stockpiling this wealth, seemed hollow to her. She had difficulty understanding the zeal that many of her fellow employees seemed to feel for becoming ever more successful…ever more wealthy. She found herself wondering if there would ever be a time when they would become satisfied with what they were acquiring.

The area of the company, in which she moved, while filled with very nice and sincere people, was geared towards serving only the extremely affluent members of their communities. One had to have at least $250,000 dollars (in excess of real estate holdings) to become a client of many of the specialists in this group. As a result, the employees dressed more carefully than the average banking employees would, were more concerned with appearances, and were more conversant with monetary topics than any singular group of people she had ever become acquainted with. She felt like a trout flopping around on dry land.

"Dr. Beall, I think you're right. I don't think I'll ever believe that training these employees to become super successful will feel as meaningful as helping young people find themselves did."

"That's what I thought. It's pretty heady stuff, helping kids. I'm not surprised that you are having a hard time giving it up," he replied.

Rozanne nodded in agreement of his assessment of her situation as a fresh batch of tears worked their way out of the corners of her eyes. She wiped them away with a clean tissue, which quickly became black with smeared mascara. "So what do I do about it?" she said at last.

"You have to begin to search for a new meaning for your life. You will go on a journey to find out who you really are and what you need to do with you life."

"How do I do that?"

"There are some techniques that I can teach you, like self-hypnosis, that can help."

Rozanne thought about what he said. She knew that Dr. Beall probably could teach her these things, but she had the feeling that this was a journey that she needed to undertake alone. She already had the tools she needed: a quick mind, a firm testimony of the gospel of Jesus Christ, and the love of her family. Even though she didn't say so at the moment, she knew that she wouldn't be coming back to Dr. Beall again. Now that she knew what was wrong—and she believed that he was totally correct in his assessment of her problem—her gut told her that she could figure out the answers she needed by herself with the help of the Lord. After all, he was the only one who had the true answers to this perplexing question…

Journal Entry: July 6, 1997

I've been looking for answers in my pursuit for obtaining a new meaning for my life. I'm not quite sure where to begin, but I have been reading a lot of things. I don't know if I will be with First Security for years or not. It's too soon to decide anything about that.

My current concern is about my Workman Compensation case. It's been over two months since I gave my deposition and I haven't heard anything. I'm getting anxious about it. The legal system works so incredibly slow. My attorney warned me that it might be this way. Boy, was he right!

Journal Entry: July 8, 1997

Something is wrong with me. I'm dizzy all of the time.

It started yesterday on my way home from work. I was sitting in my accustomed place on the bus, over the rear left tire. I like to sit there so I can rest my feet on the wheel well because my legs are so short. I was trying to read one of the books I have purchased to help me as I struggle to discover my meaning in life when I suddenly began to feel dizzy. I had to put the book away and hold my head, in an effort to make it stop feeling like it was going to fall off. I immediately went to bed when I got home, but it didn't help.

Stop the world, I want to get off!

Journal Entry: July 9, 1997

The dizziness is slowly getting worse. I don't understand what is happening to me. I told one of the women at work how I was feeling and she insisted that I call my doctor. I see him on Friday. Is this some type of bizarre flu?

Journal Entry: July 10, 1997

I almost died last night. No, really...I think I did.

I kept getting dizzier and dizzier. In the middle of the night, I began having the very real sensation that I was fading away. I could literally feel myself begin to slip out of my body. I shook Gary awake and asked him to give me a blessing, which he did. I know that the blessing saved my life. I know that I won't ever be able to convince anybody of that fact, but I know that it's true.

Journal Entry: July 11, 1997

I went to the doctor this morning. By the time it was time to go, I was so dizzy that I didn't dare drive a car, so Gary took the morning off from work and took me there. I began to feel desperately ill again as we waited to see the doctor and I wondered if I would make it into the doctor's office.

I was relieved when we were taken back to see him. I was surprised to learn that another doctor was substituting for my regular family physician. He had come down with the flu and the corporation had sent her to fill in.

As I told her what was happening to me, she became very alarmed. She asked me about my medications. I told her that my regular doctor had told me to go off of the Paxil because it didn't seem to be working for me anymore. It also made me gain weight.

"How much were you on?" she asked.

"60 milligrams," I answered.

"So tell me," she said, "did you go cold turkey?"

"Yes. Why? Is that important?" I replied.

She shook her head and ordered that a certain machine be brought into the room. The nurse wheeled it into the room and slipped a silver thing over the end of one of my fingers. This machine was to measure the oxygen saturation in my bloodstream, they told me. We waited to see what the results would be. I felt worse and worse.

I looked up to see the doctor's eyes grow large as she watched the results register. "Your blood is 97% saturated with Carbon Dioxide!" she exclaimed. Quickly, the nurse wheeled in an oxygen tank and they strapped me up. As I inhaled the oxygen, I began to feel better. Slowly the world stopped spinning.

The doctor explained to me that it is extremely dangerous to go cold turkey off of an anti-depressant. It seems that they change the body's system so drastically, that when I suddenly quit giving my body the high dosage of Paxil that it had become accustomed to, it began to slowly shut down. Without my knowledge, my breathing began to become so slow and shallow that my body wasn't getting the oxygen it needed to survive. It was fortunate that I came into the office when I did.

I guess that when I felt I was dying the other night, I truly was dying. Who would think that simply going off of a medication too quickly could cause that reaction? That is why they always caution patients to gradually quit taking their anti-depressants. I guess I hadn't paid close enough attention to what my doctor told me. Either that or I didn't take him seriously enough. I'll never make that mistake again. She gave me two weeks worth of Prozac and instructed me carefully how I was to wean myself off of the medication. I will follow her orders exactly.

I just remembered something else. My patriarchal blessing tells me that my life will be long enough that I will be able to fulfill every purpose the Lord has for me. I now know that is true. The Lord could have taken me home very easily that night. He chose not to. I must, I must discover what he wants me to do with my life!

Journal Entry: July 26, 1997

I'm completely off Prozac. I don't know what to do next about my medications. All of the anti-depressants seem to stop working for me after a while. They also make me gain a lot of weight. My gut is telling me that I still need to take something, but I don't know what. I'll have to do some praying about this, I guess.

Journal Entry: August 9, 1997

I have watched myself slip back down the hill again ever since I went off of the anti-depressants. I got up this morning, determined to find an answer. I didn't have a clue what to do about it, so I simply climbed into the van and started driving, not know where to go. I ended up going into a Deseret Bookstore that I have never seen before. I decided to see if I could find anything about alternative solutions. I wanted some guidance because I have been wary of them. My eye fell upon a big purple book that's published by TimeLife called, The Medical Advisor, The Complete Guide to Alternative & Conventional Treatments. I decided to buy it because TimeLife is a reputable company and I believed that it wouldn't have any crazy things that might not be safe. As I wandered around the store, my eye also was attracted to a CD by Felicia Sorenson. On a whim, I decided to buy it

I came home and read the book. It suggested that St. John's Wort might help with the depression. It's an herb. It said that this herb is a traditional depression remedy in Europe. The book warns that sometimes it gets remarkable results, and other times it doesn't work at all. I decided to try it so I went to a health food store and bought a couple of bottles. I'm going to cross my fingers.

I'm glad I got the CD. It makes me feel so peaceful when I listen to it. How nice!

Journal Entry: August 21, 1997

I'm getting tired of this flying around in airplanes. It seemed fun, at first. Now it doesn't. I think I should just take up residence at the Salt Lake International Airport. Maybe they should pay me as a chair warmer. I am quickly racking up the frequent flyer miles!

I feel like I'm never home. It looked like I would be home more on paper as I made up the training schedule, but it's not working out that way. I think it's taking a toll on my family. If I can just hang in there about six more weeks the worst of it will be over. My boss says that in the future we will not schedule me to be out of town nearly as much. Good!

Journal Entry: September 3, 1997

I went Visiting Teaching last week and had a great visit with Sarah. We were there for hours. She said something that distressed me, though. I was feeling great that day and remarked how grateful I felt to be feeling well. She got a peculiar look in her eye and said, "You know that you'll get depressed again, don't you? Once you go through a major depression, it always comes back again."

I felt my heart drop to the bottom of my stomach. I felt like I was going to throw up. It takes so much effort—almost a superhuman effort sometimes—to climb out of the pit once you are in it. It's such a tremendous relief to finally stand on the summit of that awful pit, and the thought that I may find myself down there again is excruciating. Oh, I hope it's not true for me, but I have a feeling that it is.

Heavenly Father, please don't leave me down there to perish if I should fall back in again. Please know that if I find myself there again, it will not because I want to be there. I will need all of the help you can send me to pull me back out. Please help me, Father.

Journal Entry: September 9, 1997

I find myself feeling more and more dissatisfied with my life here at First Security. It's not the job; it's a good one. It's not my fellow workers; they are nice and good people. I just can't shake off the feeling that this is not what I am supposed to be doing with my life.

The problem is that not only can't I seem to decide what to do, I can't seem to figure out what the Lord wants from me. It's that existentialist thing again.

Gary and I went to the temple last Saturday night with this in mind. The Lord told us both that I should quit and stay home. Gary said, "If I can just get a permanent job with benefits, Rozanne, you can quit. I'm willing."

Now the problem is this: We have lived in Utah since the summer of 1995. Gary has been looking for a permanent job ever since that time. He wants to get a job at Novell. That's what he has been trying to do for more than two years now. In fact, he is currently working as a temporary contract employee with another company at Novell. It's like he works for Novell without actually working for Novell. The company he works for pays well, but he has no benefits, no sick days, no vacation days. He doesn't even receive holiday pay.

I could quit. I want to quit. The spirit is telling me to quit, but Gary doesn't have benefits and we have five people in our family that take maintenance medications. If we had to pay for these medications by ourselves, it would break us. We couldn't possibly afford to buy them, especially if I am not working. Oh, I don't know what to do...

Journal Entry: September 15, 1997

Gary and I went to the temple again about our problem. We got the same answer to our question. I am supposed to quit my job. Help!

Okay, so if I quit my job what will I do?

I guess I could always teach music lessons. There aren't any piano teachers in our ward and people have been asking me about it. I guess I could pass flyers around advertising and pick up some students. It's certainly the right time of the year for that. But I think that there must be a purpose for me to come home besides teaching music lessons.

I know that the most important reason for me to come home is that my children have begun losing their sense of direction since I have been gone so much. I'm gone way, way, way too much for their good. Okay, that's a good reason to quit. My children need me at home.

But still, my heart tells me that there is more.

All right, Rozanne, if you could do anything you wanted to in the world, what would it be? Think big, Rozanne. Dream... Don't be afraid to dream...

Journal Entry: September 19, 1997

I've been meditating about my search this week. The questions I have been pondering are these: What is the reason for my life? What could the Lord possibly want from me? What should I do next?

As I've considered these things, I've tried to make myself remember everything I've ever done or experienced in my life. Then, while pondering the flood of memories that came to me, I've asked myself: What activities did I enjoy the very most? What secret dreams have I always harbored? What private aspirations have I had that are so deep that I haven't allowed myself to verbalize them out loud?

Journal Entry: September 20, 1997

Today I received a letter of notification in the mail that my Workman Compensation hearing will be November 11th. My attorney also sent me a letter telling me about it with instructions to meet with him a half of an hour before it starts to go over what will happen. feel like running away from home.

Journal Entry: September 22, 1997

I quit my job. I can't believe I did it, but it's true. This is how it happened:

I ride the bus to work on the days that I don't have to fly to other states. I have made a few friendships with some of the women on the West Jordan Express. This morning, as I rode, I began talking to one of my friends about what I have been considering. It was sort of nice to talk to her about it. She doesn't know me that well, and so she is not biased in one direction or the other.

I told her what I have been thinking about how I'd like to stay home and try my hand at writing music and books and how I'd decided that I could teach private music lessons, or even work as a temp to help ends meet. I told her what I was afraid of.

She listened to everything I had to say. Then she turned to me, looked me in the eye and said, "It sounds to me like you have your answer. Why don't you go ahead and just do it?"

I was stunned. All of a sudden it seemed so obvious, that I wondered why I had felt confused. I knew what the Lord wanted me to do. We had received the same answer on several different occasions in the temple. Maybe what the Lord wanted from us was a leap of faith. Just do what the spirit tells you to do and trust. I made up my mind there and then to do it as soon as my boss arrived that morning.

As soon as I could, I handed in my letter of resignation. I told my boss that I had enjoyed working there, but it had become too difficult for my family to have me gone so much. I told him that I believed I needed to explore different options. He was great and helped me get everything worked out. September 30th will be my last day.

I called Gary and told him what I had done. He said, "Honey, I trust you. I'll support you in any way I can. Go for it."

When it was all over and the dust had settled, I felt a tremendous weight lift from my shoulders. I believe that this lightening of spirit is my answer from the Lord. I did the right thing. I'm excited to see what the future holds for me…

Journal Entry: October 9, 1997

I've been busy. On the first day of my new life, (October 1) I began by designing a flyer to advertise my services as a private teacher. After I had it duplicated on fluorescent pink paper, I passed it around several subdivisions in the immediate area. I was delighted when the calls came in immediately. I already have enough students to buy groceries! I think I may be able to pull this off.

The best news is this: Gary has an interview for a permanent position at Novell. It seems almost too good to be true. After all of this time! We will surely be praying for this to happen for him. We need the benefits...

Journal Entry: October 23, 1997

He got it! He got it! He got it!

It has been a little more than three weeks since I took that leap of faith and quit my job. Heavenly Father told me to do it and when I did, He reached out his hand and caught us before we could fall. Gary got the job he has been praying for over two years. He starts in November. He'll have wonderful benefits—the best we've ever enjoyed—and tremendous educational opportunities.

You read stories like this in the Ensign all of the time, but I don't think that I ever believed that something like this would happen to me. Well, now I guess I can say it has.

Thank you Father, for your kind mercies towards my family.

Journal Entry: November 5, 1997

I took some money that I had saved from our income tax return last year and bought a corner desk for me to work at. I am determined that if I am going to try this thing. I am going to work hard at it. I decided that I better have the right tools to work with.

Journal Entry: November 11, 1997

I had my Workman's Compensation hearing today. What a circus!

I was really scared. I imagined that all sorts of terrible things would happen to me. I thought that I'd have to be on the stand and the district's lawyer would make it his business to tear me to shreds. I thought that he would try to paint a picture of me as a totally insane, unstable, loser. No wonder I was terrified!

That's not what happened at all.

We met with my lawyer briefly before it started. He went over with me what I might expect. He thought that I would probably be called to testify, which increased my level of anxiety. (I still get extremely anxious when I am confronted with any matter that concerns my breakdown and Southland Middle school.) We were both surprised, in the end, that it wasn't necessary. This is, as they say on television, what "went down:"

The district's attorney stood and started to argue his case with the judge. Imagine our surprise when he started out by saying, "The district acknowledges and relents the point that Mrs. Paxman's hospitalization was caused by her work conditions." When he said that, I thought that it was all over. After all, isn't the main purpose of Workman's Compensation Insurance to cover employees that have been injured on the job?

Apparently, I was wrong. How naïve I've been.

The lawyer went on to argue that, because of a single word that was added by the legislature to the Workman's Compensation law right before this happened to me, I should not be awarded damages. He admitted, once again, that my work conditions caused my breakdown. He also admitted that my case met the law in every instance, except the district was taking the position that this singular word in the law disqualified my claim.

So what is that word, you ask? You won't believe it. It's "sudden". That's it…the word, "sudden."

His position was that because what happened to me wasn't caused by a singular, "sudden" occurrence, I shouldn't have my medical bills paid.

I became confused by what was happening. My attorney whispered he'd explain everything afterward to me, so I sat back and watched the show.

My attorney stood and argued that while it was true that the circumstances that caused my breakdown began on day one of the school year, the incident with Jeff (the diabetic boy) was of severe enough nature to have caused my breakdown.

The opposing attorney begged to differ. He said that only a life-threatening occurrence, such as having a student threaten me with a knife or a gun, would qualify. (I want to know this: Wasn't Jeff's life threatened? Just what kind of life-threatening thing has to happen?) Then he went on to say, "Your Honor, it is our position that Mrs. Paxman's teaching conditions were not extreme.

The judge's back went straight up and she said, quite sharply, "You don't consider having fifty to sixty middle school students in a classroom "extreme?"

He replied, "But, your Honor, this is Utah."

Did that ever annoy her! She said, "Don't even go there!"

He turned red in the face and tried to back out of the mess he was in. He knew that he was on thin ice and so did we.

Then they talked about whether or not I needed to testify. My attorney said that we would stand by my deposition. The judge asked me if I agreed to that and I nodded at her. I didn't think that I could do a better job of describing what happened. I've read it. I believe I was able to portray how bad things were for me. The judge said that we could expect to hear her decision sometime after the first of the year.

After it was over, our attorney explained what happened. It seems that the last time the legislature met, the insurance companies convinced them to add this singular word, "sudden," into the section of the Workman's Compensation law that covers stress claims. They knew that this one word would make it almost impossible to prove that you deserve to have your medical bills paid. Since my case was clearly a precedent setting case, the judge didn't have any other cases to help her make up her mind. She would have to determine, in her own mind, if she could justify what happened to Jeff as severe and "sudden" enough to qualify. What's ironic about the whole thing is that if this had happened to me in 1995, my bills would have been promptly paid.

I asked him what would happen if I lost my case. He said, "You don't have any other recourse of action. You'll have to pay your own bills. The law has been written so tightly that employees are prevented from taking civil action against their employers in cases like this." Ugh! The district will possibly be able to get away with it. This will make them even less likely to care about their teachers' mental health. They won't care what kind of situations they put them in.

I told my lawyer that I don't know how that other lawyer and the people at the insurance company and the school district can sleep at night. Right is right and wrong is wrong and someday they will be accountable for what happened to me. I'll work on forgiving them, but I am extremely concerned about what will happen to other teachers now.

I don't know what the judge will decide, but I guess I'll just have to accept what happens, no matter what it is, won't I?

Journal Entry: November 15, 1997

When my friend was here yesterday, she began telling me of some abusive situations she has lived through in her life. It made me feel so bad…so hurt for her…so hurt for myself, as I remembered what the abuse I suffered caused me to go through over the years.

I don't know why I keep winding up with friends that have been abused as children. They are all good Latter-day Saint women that come from, supposedly, sound homes. They were raised in the gospel, and yet, they have experienced various levels of mental, physical, and sexual abuse. It makes me want to cry for the suffering of those innocent children that are, even now, being hurt in this terrible way.

As I meditated in this manner, the faces of my dear friends who have experienced this hurt during their lifetime kept flashing before my eyes. At last, desperate to put some of my feeling into words, I picked up my notebook and pen and wrote a song, which I have called "Don't Hurt Our Children."

I finished the song late last night and then waited with nervous anticipation to play it for my friend. I was so anxious for her to hear it, that I called her early this morning and told her that I had a gift for her. Then I sang the song over the telephone. When I was finished I waited, breathlessly, for her reaction. The phone was totally quiet. I worried that I might have offended her, but then, as I listened closer, I could hear her sniffling on the other end of the phone. She was crying.

I was wondering something yesterday as I wrote the song. Has anyone ever done a survey to see just how many women that experience major depression during her lifetimes experienced some form of abuse?

Journal Entry: November 16, 1997

I keep having nightmares lately. I don't know what to do about them.

"Help me! Help me!

Rozanne walked over to the edge of the dark crevice that opened dangerously in the center of the dry, flat plain. She didn't want to get too close. She was afraid of heights.

As she drew closer to the edge, she could see hands stretching up, and could hear the frantic voices of the individuals whose identities were lost in the darkness of the black crack in the earth. Before she could extend her hand, she looked up to see a pair of freshly scrubbed exuberant missionaries in white short-sleeved shirts rush to danger's edge to pull a pair of hands to the surface. When the feet of the exhausted man stood on solid ground once more, he threw his arms around the closer of the two young men, and sobbed with relief.

Rozanne looked to her right to see a group of people pulling with all their might on the hands of another person who was down in the crevice. They lined up, their arms firmly around the waist of the person ahead of them in line, and were straining at the difficult task they were attempting. Finally, they succeeded. The young woman arrived on the surface, her dirty face filled with joy over her narrow escape from disaster.

Then Rozanne looked across the crack. She could see other people rushing to the aide of those individuals who were still struggling to get to the surface. She was surprised to see that behind several of the rescuers, angels were pulling from behind in an effort to save all those people who wanted to be saved. It was a daunting task, but everyone at the surface was toiling with all of his or her might.

Rozanne decided to look down in the hole. She crawled carefully over to the edge, got down on her stomach so that she'd feel safer, and peered down into the darkness. In a moment, she was able to focus on the face of someone who was struggling up the craggy sides to the top. She gasped with recognition. She was staring into the same panic-stricken eyes she met every morning in the mirror.

Journal Entry: November 22, 1997

I have been feeling down this last week. I fell into the pit again. The pit gets shallower each time I fall into it and I get better at scaling the tough, rocky walls to the top again. I am learning how to call out for help and time and time again the Lord either extends his mighty arm to pull me out again, or he sends someone to help me. I am thankful for this.

I keep thinking about a dream I keep having. It's the one about the dark crevice and the rescuers. We shouldn't have to be here alone, struggling along, without the help of friends, neighbors, and family to help us. If we are in the position to help someone else, we should eagerly rush to the edge to reach out and pull willing hands to safety. Isn't this what missionary work is all about? Isn't this what temple work is all about? Isn't this what home teaching and visiting teaching is all about?

I now believe that I understand, for the first time, what the purpose of the church is all about. It is rescuing those souls, with the help of the Lord, that long for the loving arms of heaven to embrace them in the safety of the true Church of Jesus Christ. Oh, how I long to be part of it all.

Yesterday, I was feeling so sad. I rested on my bed and wrote the words, which I set to music. I call the song "Sad, Sad Lady." This morning, when a friend came to pick me up to go to the temple, I played it for her. She cried. Why do my songs keep having this effect on everybody?

Journal Entry: December 1, 1997

I wrote a humorous, light song called I Just Want To Fit In/Be Noticed last night. The music is funny, too. It makes me laugh.

Isn't that the way life is? It's a constant struggle between the two opposing forces inside us. One part of us fiercely longs to be like everybody else, to fit in, while the other side pulls just as hard the other way, longing to be noticed and appreciated.

My mom called last night. She said that she has had my name in the temple and Matthew 10:39 keeps coming to her as being the answer to my problems. I looked it up. This is what Christ teaches in this verse, "He that findeth his life shall lose it, and he that loseth his life for my sake shall find it." My heart tells me that mom is right. My soul tells me that Christ is right. I need to lose myself in service, but my mind doesn't want to accept it. I feel a battle begin to rage inside even as I write this. I guess I'll have to pray about it…

Journal Entry: Tuesday, December 15, 1997

I feel like such a fake—writing all of these songs about Christ while this illness keeps me so far away from him. I'm in so much pain that it feels hard to breathe, to think, to be. I want to be alone, and yet I don't want to be alone. I want someone to talk to me and yet, I can't hold up a conversation. I just want to curl up in a ball, or put a blanket over my head, or get in a closet…

I am getting so tired…so very tired of the struggle to keep going…to live. The war rages on inside me almost continually. I'm proud that I haven't succumbed to temptation yet, but it's getting so hard to keep climbing out of the pit over and over again. I thought I was better. I really thought that I was better.

How did I get back here and how do I get out again?

The kids are arguing. I can hardly stand the physical pain the sound of their bickering voices causes me to feel. I'd do almost anything to end it. I just long for peace.

I felt peace yesterday in the temple, but I can't stay there all of the time. Nothing really interests me.

I go shopping and just wander around looking, but nothing appeals to me. It's hard to Christmas shop this way.

I want something good to eat, but nothing tastes good or satisfies me so I'm eating terribly. I've been skipping meals for the first time in my life because it is too much trouble to find something to eat.

Last night, for the first time, I tolerated relations with Gary. I normally enjoy it, but since I feel this way nothing appeals to me. I didn't want Gary to suffer, though, because I feel like stone. That's why I did it. I think he could tell though.

Poor Gary…I wonder how long he'll be able to take it—me feeling and acting this way. How do I turn it around? Just what do I need to do to change things?

I read the scriptures. I try to pray, but praying is the hardest thing of all to do because my words get all jumbled up and confused. My thoughts go round and round. I begin thinking that I'm not making much sense. I can't get my true self's thoughts and feelings expressed. I know they are in there, somewhere, but I can't get them out.

I scare myself and I'm afraid that I'm offensive to the Lord as I struggle with this illness. I'd rather have cancer. I could understand cancer. I'm sick, but I can't find the physician that can heal me.

I get pictures in my head of me swallowing pills and just going to sleep…or cutting myself…or wrecking the car…or jumping off of the house. These images are the hardest to rid myself of. I try and try and try to shut them out, but they keep sneaking back in like a garbage can that fills back up as soon as you've emptied it.

This is the war that I'm raging—the war for my soul. This war leaves little left over for anything or anyone. I feel like I'm getting sucked down a wormhole...

Journal Entry: December 22, 1997

I used to get so much happiness—or maybe it was just thrills—out of acquiring things. I'd think that if I could just get this or that, then I'd be happy. I would spend a lot of time—especially during this time of year—thinking about what I'd like to get.

As I got older, I found myself spending money and effort to acquire belongings until finally—just like a kids who eats too much candy—I felt satiated and "sort of sick." Everything that I thought brought me happiness was really hollow (like wearing nice clothing, having a nice home, playing first chair in the orchestra, performing, driving a snappy little car). Even the things that I wanted that are truly good to have—like children—I think that I wanted them for the wrong reasons. I wasn't thinking about them. I was only thinking about me. How did I grow up and stay so self-centered for so many years? Now that I want to change this sad fact about myself, I am at a loss as to how to do it.

Once I realized that what I previously wanted was of no value, I was left feeling empty and hollow. I knew that I didn't feel any happiness acquiring the things I used to enjoy, so any effort I make to try to go back to where I was before my breakdown, is pointless. I realize that I don't want to recapture the shallow happiness of my former self. I want desperately to come out of this experience transformed into a newer, better me.

As I have struggled, I have gradually come to realize that what I long for most of all is to feel the love of God in my heart and to experience the peace that comes with this love. I want to feel it throughout every pore of my mortal body. I want to feel the love of God so totally, that I am free to allow it to overflow from me and spill onto those around me. I believe that if I can feel His love this much (I think that this feeling I desire must be charity...) then I will be able to become God's agent for good and be able to bless the lives of others. I think I may finally understand why the angel told Nephi that the fruit of the tree of life represents the love of God. This feeling, to know God's love, truly is the most precious and desirable of all."

I want the days of self-centeredness and self-interest to be lost forever. There is no true peace or happiness in that dreary land. I have decided that Christ is right. I must lose myself to find myself. So here is how I have begun my quest...

Last Saturday I went down to a care center that is only a few blocks from my home. I wanted to do something for someone just to be kind. I haven't told anyone about this, nor do I intend to. I want this thing to be different. The old me would have told others in order to receive a pat on the back for doing something nice, but I want to start doing things for other people to try to earn the gift of charity.

I know how it feels to be alone. I know how it feels to be so lonely you think that your heart will break. Now that I've experienced this emotion, I don't like the idea that there may be people out there that need me and I'm not doing anything about it. I'm sure that the Lord tried to get someone to help me during my darkest days, but for one reason or another, they ignored his promptings. I shudder to think how many times I may have done the same thing. Hopefully, I won't let this happen again.

I entered the care center that I thought, at first, was a home for the elderly. I was dismayed when I realized my mistake. This center specialized in the care and treatment of adult Down's Syndrome patients. I felt scared and wanted to leave, but the spirit whispered to me, "These are my children, too," so I proceeded. I asked the attendant at the desk if I could see someone who doesn't get many visitors and he took me to meet a girl named Jenny.

Jenny was sitting by the door watching out the window, waiting for someone to take her home. The attendant told me that her "someone" would never arrive. Her lonely vigil, with suitcase in hand, was doomed for failure.

Jenny can hardly talk, but she seems to understand some things. I drew a lot of pictures in her notebook, sang Christmas songs to her, and then I talked to her about the holiday season. Some other patients heard my singing and moved closer so they could hear the cheerful melodies.

When I left, Jenny kissed me on the cheek. I can't forget the feel of her soft lips on my face. It was an expression of innocent love and gratitude. I keep thinking about Jenny and I want to go back.

Jenny seemed so keenly alone. I don't think I've ever experienced the level of loneliness that she wore in her expression when I first spotted her. It haunts me. I think I'll go and get her some new markers and a notebook and take them to her.

I'm going to keep this experience as my very own little private secret. Maybe in time, when I've figured things out, I'll take my little kids there. I don't want them to grow up as self-centered and selfish as I am. Maybe I can find a way to prevent that from happening.

I pray that the Lord will show me the way. I sincerely want to become more like Christ. I think that maybe I don't have friends because I'm not very friendly. People don't want to hear me talking about myself. They want me to be interested in them. Oh, I have so much to learn!

Journal Entry: December 22, 1997

I went to K-Mart and put together a gift bag of things for Jenny. We don't have very much money right now, but it was important to me to do it. I bought two different sizes of markers, a couple of notebooks (she seems to prefer these), a large school box to put them in. I also bought her a candy bar. I hoped that will be all right. I wasn't sure how the center feels about candy…

When I got to the desk and asked for Jenny, she was walking down the hall towards me. She squealed and ran over to me and gave me a great big hug. She was so happy to see me.

There was a different attendant at the desk. She was a cross old lady, who appeared to be in her late sixties.

She demanded, "Who are you and how do you know Jenny?"

I explained to her what happened the previous Saturday.

She looked down her nose at me and said, "We can't just have people walking off of the street and coming in here! We have to look out for our patients. People may come in here and try to take advantage of them. Their parents wouldn't like that."

That was hard—to have her act like I was a deviant just because I wanted to do something nice. I explained to her that I had been a schoolteacher (thinking that if she knew that, she'd believe that I am trustworthy) and that I just wanted to do something nice for someone who needed it. She was extremely suspicious. She said, "The only way you are allowed to come here is with the prior approval of the social worker. She'll have to do a background check on you."

I told her that I would be happy to do anything they felt was necessary. I gave her my phone number to give to the social worker. I told her that I would like to volunteer at the center. She acted like I was crazy. I doubt they'll ever call.

This all happened while Jenny was standing by me, holding my hand, grinning so happily. It was pathetic.

At last, the woman agreed to let me give Jenny her gift and we went to the group room, where many other patients were sitting. Jenny opened her gifts with as many squeals of joy as one hears from a whole family of small children on Christmas morning. She was thrilled. I drew her some more pictures, and sang some Christmas songs. The other patients gathered round us, with requests for pictures of Santa Claus and songs they knew and loved. They were happy to have me there. I wish I could go back, but I know that I won't be able to. I guess I'll just have to find something else nice to do...

Journal Entry: December 29, 1997

Today was a good day. We got a lot done around here. We cleaned up and put away the Christmas decorations. It's always fun to put them out after Thanksgiving, but amazingly, it feels like such a relief to put them away again.

Something very scary happened tonight. Julianne and I went down to the Arctic Circle on Redwood Road to get some dinner for the family. For some reason, I could not get her seatbelt to fasten. Foolishly, I decided to proceed anyway.

After I got the food, I headed north on Redwood. Suddenly, I felt a terrible headache coming on. It was hard to think. I started to make the left hand turn onto 70th South and I misjudged the distance. I rammed into the medium with the left front wheel of the truck. The force of the impact spun us around 180 degrees. We went all over the road and ended up facing the wrong direction. There were cars everywhere but, mercifully, we didn't hit anybody. What was even more amazing, Julianne was still in her seat.

It was a miracle. While we were spinning, I had the strange sensation that a giant hand had control of us. The hand kept us from getting hit by another car and it kept us from rolling over. The Lord protected us and I'm very grateful.

I'm not sure why he protected us, but I know his hand was in it and I feel blessed. If he wanted me to die, it surely could have happened tonight. Maybe my life is more important that I thought...

This experience increases my desire to try to live even better than before, as I finally believe I must have a purpose. There must be something that I, alone, am supposed to do. I wonder what it is...

Here are the gifts I gave to Christ this year that no one else knows about:

Two visits to the Care Center.

$20.00 to the ward's Christmas fund (I gave it anonymously. I know the bishop will never suspect me because he was worried about Christmas for us. How fun!)

A van full of blankets, coats, and hats to a homeless shelter

I know it's not much, but it's a start. I want to do even more.

I pray that the Lord will help me find answers to these questions.

Journal Entry: January 10, 1998

Metamorphosis: change of physical form, structure, or substance especially by supernatural means.

Metamorphic rock: rocks that have been changed through heat and pressure.

Heat and pressure...I guess I am going through a metamorphosis.

Journal Entry: January 12, 1998

I had a slight cold today so I didn't feel like doing anything. I did something I never do...I watched the Montel Williams show. I was lucky. It actually was pretty good. He had a doctor on that was talking about the power of the human heart to believe. He said that there have been scientific studies done that show that the heart actually has power to make things happen. It sounded more like faith to me, but it got me thinking. I put together a little song, which I rather like. I call it, "What the Heart Knows." The lyrics talk about the idea that the heart can see, and love, other people better than the eyes and mind can.

The last verse talks about the idea that if you hold your love to tightly to yourself and you don't let yourself love other people freely, your loving feelings shrivel up and die. On the other hand, the more freely you extend your love to others, the more love you have to give.

I think that most of us (at one time or another) have desperately wished that other people could see inside us—that they could see the true person we are and not judge us simply by our appearance. I think that there is nothing about me, physically, that would appeal to the world and yet, I am a child of God, just like everyone else. I wish I could hand people a crystal looking glass that would allow them to look at me and see the beautiful spirit Father created. I wish I could carry this looking glass around with me and use it to see other people clearly, as well. Maybe if we tried to look at each other with the heart instead of the eyes…

Journal Entry: January 15, 1998

As I read the scriptures I keep stumbling over two things. One is the many, many times Christ tells us to knock and he'll open to us, pray and we'll receive and so on. There are more than fifteen references to these promises in the standard works. He must mean what he says. That is probably why he has repeated it so much…He knows how thickheaded we can be sometimes.

The other thing I keep stumbling onto is the story of the woman with a blood disease that manages to touch Christ's hem through the press of the crowd and is healed because of her faith. In fact, every time I open my scriptures, the book falls open to this story. Maybe I'm supposed to do something with these ideas…

Journal Entry: January 18, 1998

I have been pondering the scriptures I mentioned in the last journal entry. I finally came to the conclusion that I should try to write a song about it. I came up with a song about the woman which I called, "The Blessings of the Kingdom."

As I wrote the song, the thought kept coming to me that I am very much like the woman in the story. I have an illness that I need the Savior's help with. I have come to the decision that although the medication and therapy was absolutely necessary, ultimately it will be Christ who heals me of this affliction. I've got to muster up the same kind of faith she had. I've got to believe his promises to us. I'm knocking, Lord…I'm knocking…

Journal Entry: February 5, 1998

I got feeling kind of blue tonight. I received the judge's decision about my Workman's Compensation claim. She had to rule against me because she just couldn't justify that what happened to Jeff could be classified as a severe and "sudden" incident. She added a statement at the end of her decision though, that said that this decision was not satisfactory to her. She wanted to rule in my favor. She feels that I deserved to win, but that stupid, stupid word in the law prevents her from ruling the way she wanted to. Oh, well…

Naturally, her decision made me feel bad, although I've been expecting it to turn out this way. I began feeling depressed, worrying about what would happen now. Luckily, I've gained some coping skills and I was smart about what I did. I asked Gary for a blessing. I'm trying to make myself ask Gary for a blessing when I first get depressed, rather than to let myself slide down to the bottom before it becomes painfully obvious that I need one.

After the blessing was over, I got into our comfortable king-sized waterbed and enjoyed the most calm, peaceful feeling that I believe I've ever experienced. I was floating on warm water, and felt that my spirit was enveloped in warm, calm spiritual water. It occurred to me that this feeling may be the living water that Christ speaks of.

I began hearing a beautiful melody and words. I jumped out of bed and went downstairs to my office and began working. In just a few, short, hours, I had finished a lovely song. I believe it is very, very special. It's title is "Calm Waters."

It is possible to change. It is possible to start living outside yourself and caring for other people. It is possible to become what you were meant to be.

Journal Entry: April 12, 1998

I think I have been given an answer to my prayers today. It came from an unexpected source. A fresh-faced returned missionary gave his homecoming talk in Sacrament Meeting this afternoon. It was a good talk, but what struck me the most was when he began telling us about his experiences with living the mission rules. It seems that he had struggled with them, at first, but as he persisted in becoming more exact in his observance of the rules, his ability to do his work increased.

This thought electrified me—down to my very core. I don't recall the rest of his talk at all. The spirit just keep telling me, "That's what you need to do…That's what you need to do. You're on a mission for the Lord, and you need to observe missionary rules as much as it is possible, under your circumstances."

I asked the Lord what mission he was referring to and he answered, "You will know in time."

I felt the warmth of the Holy Ghost envelop me with the truthfulness of these words. I felt that I was finally on the path the Lord intends for me. I felt that someday, all of my suffering would bring solace and comfort to others.

I wondered about the missionary rules…what the Lord meant for me to do. The spirit answered, "You need to go to bed early and get up early. You need to study the scriptures at length, every day. You need to pray often. You need to separate yourself from the evil influences of the world that you are so attracted to."

I asked, "What influences?"

The spirit answered, "Television and movies…These things are your downfall. It is through these things that you allow Satan to come into your life. You need to be extremely careful what you watch."

That's going to be hard for me. I do so love to lose myself in a good television show or a movie, but I know the Lord is right. I'm noticing that it's always after a period of intense television and movie indulgence, that I get depressed. Then, when I'm depressed, I want to watch them even more. I guess I was right when I was in the hospital. TV is my drug of choice, and I've got to break the habit.

I feel an excitement that I haven't felt in years. I feel like I'm finally on my way.

Journal Entry: April 26, 1998

I had a special experience today. I opened my scriptures to read during the sacrament and the book fell open to Colossians 2: 6, "As ye have therefore received Christ Jesus the Lord, so walk ye in him;" I kept pondering this scripture throughout the afternoon.

After dinner, I went into our bedroom so that I could be alone. I opened my scriptures and they fell open to this verse again. As I meditated on Paul's words, the thought came to me that I need Christ's help so that I can "walk in him." I said out loud, "Lord, walk with me. I need your help." When I heard my own words, I was a struck with a powerful feeling. I looked back at the page and as I did, I began hearing a melody being sung to the words, "Walk with me, take my hand, lead me ever to the Promised Land…"

I knew that the spirit was going to give me a song so I went down to my office. In just a short time I had it. It's amazing to me how the spirit works. Sometimes, I receive a song that is already so beautiful and pure that I don't have to change a single thing. Other times, I have to sweat and labor over every syllable and note. I have to edit and rearrange to make the song satisfactory. This song, which I am calling, "Walk With Me," is one of the special ones.

Journal Entry: May 3, 1998

I have been busily writing songs…lots of songs…all kinds of songs. In the past six months, I have written songs about Christ and my experiences with him. I have written funny songs about life, and my view of it. I have written songs about my past. I have written choir arrangements, instrumental arrangements, orchestral arrangements, duets, trios, and just about anything else you can imagine. Writing this music has been very cathartic. I find that I am able to express my feelings and emotions better through the marriage of lyrics and music than I can with words alone.

Journal Entry: May 10, 1998

I've had a very unusual day. This afternoon, a neighbor called up and falsely accused one of our children. I know the accusation was false because I called the individuals involved and found out the details for myself. My son was supposed to have hurt another boy, but the boy told me himself that it didn't happen. They were fooling around and some other kids that saw it didn't understand what had happened. I called back the neighbor and told him what I had learned. He said that it didn't matter, he thought my son was always in trouble.

I went in my bedroom and cried. I felt so tired of being misjudged. I have felt that way so often. In fact, I've felt that way most of my life. I felt alone and misunderstood. Gary and I try so hard to be good parents, but it seems sometimes, that no matter how hard you try, there are always people ready and happy to point fingers at you and tell you that you are failing.

The longer I thought about what had happened, the worse I felt. I thought, "Why can't people like us? What is so bad about us? Why can't we be accepted? We are trying so very hard to do what is right."

As I continued feeling sorry for myself, I heard the bedroom door open, then close again. I wondered what that was all about, but I chose to ignore it. I began to feel like the weight of the countless times throughout my life when I have felt alone, friendless, or misunderstood, came crashing down on my head. Just as I started to feel that I would be lost in a pit of despair, I heard the Lord say in my mind, "Rozanne, I understand what you're feeling. Remember, I was never understood during my life. I was even betrayed by my closest friends. Now I have something for you. Get your notebook."

I got my notebook and began to write what came to me. The beauty and power of the words amazed me.

As I wrote the words down one line, "give me the ones, for whom there's no room at the inn," immediately jumped out at me. I felt like the Savior was telling me that he understands how I feel. He didn't even have a decent place to be born. He was among those people who are not popular, who are not understood. Even among his followers, most of them didn't understand what he was trying to tell them. The multitudes followed him, but not for the spiritual healing he offered them. They followed him to be healed physically and to have their hungry bellies satisfied. He wanted them to open their eyes and hear his words, but they just couldn't seem to understand what he was telling them.

It makes me feel better to know that he understands me. Somehow, I don't ever think I'll feel quite as bad as I used to about not feeling accepted. I know that I'll probably always walk on the fringe of popular society, courting its favor, but remain destined never to walk its halls.

I have decided to sing this song on Fast Sunday as my testimony. That will seem peculiar to some people, but I know the Lord will understand. I'm able to express, through my music, what I'm not able to communicate when I speak. I'm learning so much as I travel this long road to becoming whole.

Journal Entry: June 1, 1998

The financial pressure is starting to get to me. I am earning only a small percentage of what I brought in when I was working for First Security. I came home because I believed it was what the Lord wanted me to do. It was a leap of faith and the Lord blessed us for it.

I have been trying to cut corners everywhere I can. I shop at food outlets. I buy our clothes at the second-hand stores. Our only entertainment comes from the public library. I walk everywhere I can. There are no luxuries like dentist appointments, or eye exams in this house. Some days, the worry and fear that I have that I won't be able to make ends meet and that I won't be able to feed the children or pay the bills fills me with so much dread that often I can taste bile as it tries to find its way to the surface.

It's getting harder every day. Our house payment is high, even though this is an ordinary little house. I'm terrified that if some disaster happened, we would be financially devastated. There are many, many weeks that we have to live off of food storage because I have chosen to pay our tithing, rather than have the money to go food shopping. I go around, with a tight feeling in my stomach, worrying…worrying…worrying…Father in Heaven…We need help.

I wrote a song, which I call "An Answered Prayer," about the struggle that I sometimes experience as I try to pray. I want so desperately to improve the level of my communication with the Lord. It's improving, but I still have so very far to go. The Lord has let me know, quite firmly, that I need to pray twice a day on my knees. It's helping my efforts to obey his will.

As I worked on the song, I almost felt like I was being choked. I decided that, maybe, it isn't a good song, so I put it away and didn't play it for anyone for quite a while.

At last, I decided that I should share it with someone and I played it for a friend, almost apologetically. Her reaction shocked me. She loved it and she told me that it's special. I've been thinking about it and have decided that maybe the choked, depressed feeling I was having while working on it was the adversary trying to get me to stop. Maybe it's going to be important to someone someday. Who knows? No one but the Lord can answer that question.

Journal Entry: June 30, 1998

A few days ago, after fasting and attending the temple for guidance, I received a special message from the spirit. I was told many things that I should do. It came so fast to me in my mind that I had to get out a piece of paper and a pen to write it down, so I wouldn't forget what I was hearing. I will do as I was instructed, not knowing why, because I trust that the Lord has his purposes, even though I may not understand now.

I believe that the last thing I wrote down was the most important. He said, "Pray always for my help and I will give it to you. I will send angels to attend thee: one to the right hand and one to the left—one to go before you as you go and one to walk behind you to keep you safe. Go, my daughter, go and do your work."

This gives me a sense of strength, especially since I believe that I know who my angels are; they are my deceased family members. Who else would love and care for me as much as they do? Who else would believe that I am able to do whatever the Lord wants me to do? Who else would want to watch over me? I believe that when we need extra help—to complete a mission, or to resist evil, or to be kept safe—that the Lord sends us our family members to help us.

I believe that during the times I felt so alone…during the times when I felt like I must die…during the times that I felt that my life didn't matter, the Lord sent my family to help me. It was during the times of extreme temptation that they stood by me to buoy me up. I didn't know that they were there then, but I do now. The Lord was there, the Holy Ghost was there, and my family was there. I know this because I'm alive today.

I know something else—something that I wish everyone who was ever depressed enough to think of dying could know.

A few months ago I was feeling sad and guilty about the suicidal feelings I had experienced. I thought that the Lord must be very angry with me for feeling that way. As I continued to think these things, a thought entered my mind as forcefully as if someone had shouted it in my ear. I heard the Lord say, in my mind, "Rozanne, I am not angry with you. I am proud of you. You have experienced a level of temptation that few people ever know, and yet, you have resisted that temptation. I am proud of you, my beloved daughter."

How happy I was! How relieved I was! How thankful I was that I had resisted the temptations I had faced. It has given me strength, so much strength, to know that those suicidal thoughts didn't originate in me. They came from the evil one.

Now, when the suicidal thoughts pop into my mind they are much, much easier to disperse with, because I know that they come from outside of me. I didn't think them originally.

I have learned that when a suicidal thought enters my mind, I don't have to entertain it. I can tell Satan that, in the name of the Savior, Jesus Christ, he must leave me alone. When I do this, I feel him leave. It's a physical sensation. I can't explain it, but how very grateful I am to know that I can make him leave me alone for a while.

I want everyone to know that they have this right, as well. I want them to know that they can make Satan leave with Christ's help. I want them to know that suicidal thoughts are temptations…temptations that they can resist, with the Lord's help. I want them to know that if it gets too hard to resist these temptations by themselves, that they should ask for help. They should get a blessing. They should call a suicide hot line. They should call 911. They should go to see their doctor. They should cry out for help.

They must get help. Their life is valuable and they are loved. They don't have to feel alone.

Journal Entry: July 18, 1998

I want to be able to help other people. I'm tired of having to need help. I used to be so self-sustaining and self-reliant. I've been learning many lessons since my breakdown, one of which is humility. I've had to learn to accept gifts and help from others. It's been hard.

Journal Entry: July 25, 1998

This week was fun! I decided that I'd had enough worries for a while and so I took my little kids down to St. George to visit mom and dad. James and Stephen had to work, so they stayed home with Gary. Mom and Dad had just purchased a used travel van, with cushy seats, and a television and a videocassette player. They wanted to go on a little trip and they wanted me to drive them.

We went through the tunnel that cuts through a mountain in Zion's Canyon, so that we could drive over to Bryce's Canyon. I honked the horn when we were in the long, dark tunnel and the kids squealed with laughter. After we ate a picnic lunch in Bryce's Canyon, we drove north for a while before crossing the mountain to Cedar Breaks and driving back down the other side into Cedar City. After we had eaten dinner in Cedar City, we drove back home to St. George. Mom bought me a new T-shirt in Cedar Breaks, the first new one I've had in a long time.

As I drove, Dad sat in the passenger seat and talked to me. He asked me why I was so worried all of the time. I told him what was going on. He was amazed to hear what our house payment is and that it isn't possible to rent a similar house for less money in the Salt Lake Valley. He said, "Grandma, Rozanne and Gary need to move to Holden and live in the house you inherited from your father."

I about wrecked the van.

Mom didn't know what to say, either, for a while. But after we talked about it, we decided that maybe it would be a good idea.

It's a frightening thought. I'd be going home. I never, in my wildest imaginations, thought that someday I would be living in Millard County again. I ran away from there as a youth. What would it be like to live there as an adult? Do I want to do it?

On the way home from St. George, I stopped by the family home in Holden and walked around. There's a lot of property around the house that needs to be taken care of. Can I do it?

Do I want to do it? I started to sweat and felt my head swim, so I climbed back into our van and drove home.

I told Gary tonight about Mom and Dad's offer. He didn't even seem surprised. He said that the thought has been popping into his mind, ever since my aunt died and left the house empty, that we'd be living there someday. I don't know about this…I just don't know…

Journal Entry: August 3, 1998

I had a dream tonight. I was walking through the house in Holden. I kept saying, "There has to be another bedroom here…There has to be another bedroom." I looked everywhere for it. I looked in the kitchen cupboards, in the closets, under the beds and finally, I found it. It was in the attic. I believe the attic has enough headroom to make another bedroom up there. Maybe it would work…

Journal Entry: August 7, 1998

I've got to make up my mind what we're going to do. If we are going to move to Holden, we've got to do it soon. I'll have to go down to Holden next week to enroll the kids in school. I feel pushed…

Journal Entry: August 8, 1998

I went to the temple today. Gary and I have been fasting about what to do. I got the strong feeling that we should move to Holden. Gary agrees. So Holden, ready or not...here we come...

Journal Entry: August 12, 1998

I'm exhausted. We just spent three of the most miserable days scrapping wallpaper off of the kitchen and dining room and followed by hours of painting. We have to get this house ready to sell. There were several layers of paper to peel off. Even the top layer, which was supposed to be dry-strippable, had to be scraped off. Little Julianne was such a trooper. She worked for two days, pulling the vinyl tops off of the paper. I didn't know she had it in her.

James and his friend helped me paint. I have worked so hard that I feel like bawling, but it's done. Gary will have to finish what's left around here. The kids and I leave for Holden tomorrow morning. We have to enroll them in school. By the end of next week, the children and I will be living there permanently.

Journal Entry: August 22, 1997

We're living in Holden now. It's been a hard week for me. I felt such peace when the children and I were here last week to enroll them in school. I felt a sense of peace that I haven't experienced in years. Then, at the beginning of this week, we went back up to West Jordan to pack up our necessities to move them down here.

After a couple of days in that house, I got such a dark, ugly feeling—so depressed again—that Gary made me bring the kids down here earlier than we had originally planned. It's difficult to explain what it was like. I began to feel intense doom and gloom. I think that I was feeling that way because the thought that we didn't have to move kept coming into my mind. I'd hear, "You're crazy. You don't have to move down there. Look—you have a nice home here in West Jordan. Your children have friends. They're doing well in school. You don't have to move."

The more those thoughts kept going through my mind, the worse I felt. Finally, I told Gary what was going on and he made me leave right then. It was so hard to do that I actually turned around, after driving south a couple of blocks, and went back to the house. Gary saw me drive back in and marched up to the truck window. I rolled it down only to hear him give me my orders. He said, not too patiently I must add, "Rozanne leave! You'll feel better once you're there. Just wait and see…"

He was right. The closer I got to Holden, the better I felt. By the time I had pulled into town, a light, buoyant spirit had replaced the dark, ugly one I had been experiencing in West Jordan. I believe that is a pretty strong indicator that the decision to move here is the correct one. I think that Satan must have been trying to make me doubt our decision. The move down here must be a critical one for our family, but I guess I'll just have to be patient and let life show me why.

I'm happy about one thing, in particular. After we get matters arranged with the West Jordan home, I won't have to work at all, if I don't want to. This will be the first time in years and years that I will have that choice. Our expenses will be so much lower here, that Gary will be able to support us on his own. Anything that I bring in will be able to go towards our future and the children's missionary fund and educational fund. Hooray!

Journal Entry: September 16, 1998

I saw something on the Oprah Winfrey show today that struck a nerve. She was talking about a book she read called, "Simple Abundance, A Daybook of Comfort and Joy", which was written by Sarah Ban Brethnach. Sarah recommends that everyday you write down five things that you are grateful for. She says that after two months of writing these things down everyday, you won't be the same person. Expressing your gratitude opens your eyes to what you have and you become more content. It also opens you to receive more blessings. Oprah said it worked for her. The scriptures in D&C 59 about gratitude came to my mind as she talked. Verses 15 and 16 of that section read, "And inasmuch as ye do these things with thanksgiving, with thankful hearts and countenances, not with much laughter, for this is a sin, but with a glad heart and a cheerful countenance…verily I say, that inasmuch as ye do this, the fulness of the earth is yours."

I have another journal that I started a while ago and then abandoned. I think I'll turn it into a gratitude journal and try the experiment. After all, isn't that what Alma and Amulek recommended the Zoramites do when they were learning about faith? You have to try it, hoping that it is true and then you will be able to judge for yourself by the outcome if it is so. Well, here I go…

Journal Entry: September 23, 1998

I choose to be happy from this time forward. I choose to enjoy today, this minute.

Journal Entry: October 7, 1998

I have discovered another key in my search for wellness. I think that I have heard this before, but maybe I'm finally ready to believe it now. This is the key: "The thought process itself is the key to exercising faith."

I guess I better tell where I learned this important fact. I have had a little book by Grant Von Harrison entitled, "Drawing of the Powers of Heaven," for a long time. When I was in West Jordan that last day, I went downstairs to look for some papers and I spotted this little book sitting on top of one of the many stacks of books that we own. I had forgotten that we had it. The spirit told me to take it with me. I obeyed, but didn't do anything with it for a while.

I just started to read it last week. You can't just read it straight through. It's a book that you need to read, stop and meditate about what you are learning, then answer the questions and the do the exercises. I had determined that I was going to work very hard, since I've moved to Holden, at progressing spiritually. I decided to increase the effort I have been making ever since the time I decided to follow missionary rules. When I spotted the little blue book again, it occurred to me that perhaps something in it would help me grow spiritually.

I have been struck by the many truths I find in it. But the most important thing I have learned during my study, is the new understanding I have gained of how faith actually works. Faith has always been sort of an enigma to me. I knew I needed it. I knew I wanted it. But I just wasn't sure how to go about getting more of it.

For the first time in my life I know what to do. I learned that in order to increase your faith, you have to work at controlling your thoughts. Brother Von Harrison talks a lot about it. That's what Joseph Smith taught, too. He said in the Lectures on Faith that when you are working by faith, you are working by mental exertion.

Brother Von Harrison teaches that we need to examine our thoughts, determine if they help or hurt you, then replace negative thoughts with thoughts that will help you. I know that it seems, on the surface, to be so simple...almost too simple. But the spirit is telling me that it is true. I believe that it is true.

As I've been meditating about what I read in this book, I have been examining what has happened to me during the past several years. I think I can see that if I had just known this truth before, and if I had been actively pursuing a program of controlling my thoughts, I wouldn't have experienced a nervous breakdown. I would have had the tools I needed to control my thoughts, thereby controlling my emotions.

Journal Entry: October 10, 1998

Brother Von Harrison recommends that you write down what your righteous desires are and the steps you will take to accomplish your goals. He also recommends that you write down what help you will need from the Lord, in order to accomplish your goals, and the commitments you will make to the Lord, in order to qualify for your desires to be realized. He then tells you to pray to the Lord and submit your plan for his approval. If the spirit tells you that there are things about your plan that need revising, then make the changes.

I've never thought about taking these steps before. I'm going to think about what I would like to do and then submit my own plan to the Lord. I wish, I wish, I wish that I'd known about this before.

I've been trying to control my thoughts. I've been memorizing hymns to sing. Brother Von Harrison recommends that you try to think about righteous things during the times that you would normally let your mind wander, like when you are getting ready in the morning or when you are driving in the car. I've memorized all of the verses to the hymn, "How Firm a Foundation." It gives me such a sweet feeling when I am singing it to myself as I am working around the house, or driving to Fillmore and back. I remember now that Boyd K. Packer recommends memorizing hymns. I can vaguely remember a filmstrip we were shown in Mutual about our thoughts. Why didn't I pay closer attention? I wish I had been doing this before. It really works!

By the way, the gratitude journal experiment is fantastic. My eyes have been opened. How could I have walked around all of these years so blind to the beauty of the world around me and the wonders of the many blessings the Lord has given me? I feel so grateful to have been given this idea. Hey! I can write that in my gratitude journal!

Journal Entry: October 13, 1998

I took the little kids to St. George last weekend and went to the temple twice. I had a good experience. Gary and I fasted that the Lord would bless us in the matter of the West Jordan home. I was also fasting about the goals I have set.

After the last session, I felt the spirit strongly. My chest almost felt like it was on fire. After I had silently prayed, I heard in my mind that the Lord has something special for me to do. I was told not to watch television and movies. I would need to make this sacrifice to be able to get my work done. I was told that this was important for two reasons: 1. They waste my time. 2. They take me backward spiritually and undo the progress I make.

Why are these things such a temptation for me? I do well for a while, and then I give in to tiredness or boredom and watch them again. I know the Lord is right. I've got to make the sacrifice. How can I learn to control my thoughts if I am dumping bad thoughts back in again while I am watching television?

Journal Entry: October 21, 1998

Last night I went visiting teaching and by the time I got home, the kids were so starving I just threw a pizza in the oven and we gobbled it up. I'm ashamed to admit that I watched about an hour of a yucky movie before Julianne brought me to my senses. I just can't watch television at all. When will I learn?

It is such a struggle to constantly monitor what I'm thinking and saying, but I'm trying to do this. I can tell how important it is. If I can just get a hold on it permanently, I can overcome depression, discouragement, and the other tools of Satan by relying instead, on my faith in Jesus Christ and the influence of the Holy Ghost. I am noticing that the harder I try and the longer I am able to maintain my vigilance, the closer to the Lord I feel.

Julianne begged me to allow her to take my porcelain doll, the one with the sad face I called Rozanne, into school for show-and-tell. I was hesitant, but it seemed so important to her that I finally broke down and allowed it.

When she returned home, her face was as white as a ghost and I knew that something bad had happened. She accidentally dropped "Rozanne" on her head and the doll's face broke off. Julianne started to cry when she told me. She felt awful about it. The funny thing is that it didn't bother me at all. I think it would have bothered me if "Rosie" had been broken, but somehow, it seemed right that Rozanne "died" like that. I don't need her anymore. The person that she reminded me of is gone and so it seems right that she is gone as well.

Journal Entry: October 26, 1998

Yesterday was a hard day. I got sick in the morning and had to come home early from church. Gary was still up in West Jordan so I had to feed and manage the kids by myself.

Gary and I both feel that we are at our limits. We haven't been able to sell the house and we've been having a problem with the title.

After I went to my room, I knelt by my bed and prayed so fervently that I wore myself out. I was crying and pleading to the Lord for help. When I was spent, I climbed into bed. Right before I fell asleep, I heard the spirit say, "I love you, Rozanne. I love you. I love you…"

This morning, as I was studying the scriptures, I began to meditate and I briefly fell asleep. When I woke up, I was hearing a voice sing the hymn, "When Faith Endures." The words were ringing in my head. I knew that I should get out my hymnbook and look at it.

I got out my Family Home Evening book and prepared a lesson on increasing faith. I felt so peaceful and loved. I am now working on memorizing this hymn.

I don't know how—everything is quite chaotic now—but things will work out and we will see the Lord's hand in it. He does love me. He does take notice of me.

How I wish to serve him in anyway that he'll let me. I want, most of all, to cleanse the inner vessel and become pure of heart—to be worthy (through the Atonement, of course) of his confidence and attention of me.

Journal Entry: October 27, 1998

Last night Gary was home. We had a real family dinner and then, together, we taught the Family Home Evening lesson. It was good for all of us. The lesson on faith went well and the children seemed to get it.

I have such a sense of peace being here in Holden again. I told the kids last night that I felt like I had been on an extremely long journey for years and years. Now, finally, I am back home. I love living in this little house, the same little house that my beloved Grandma Stevens raised her family in. I love driving around this valley and seeing the beautiful mountain ranges that I grew up enjoying. I love walking the streets and having people I know wave at me. I love going to the stores and meeting old friends and acquaintances. I love knowing that I am related to half of the county. I love knowing that all of the old hurts of my youth are forgotten and forgiven. I feel whole.

Last night, before we went to bed, I looked at Gary and began to cry. But my tears were not tears of sorrow this time. My tears were tears of joy. He laughed in delight to see me so happy. Finally, at long last, I have experienced true joy. How grateful I am to the Lord for his help as I have walked this long agonizing journey. I know that I'll probably have hard times again. That's to be expected. I probably will have periods of depression, but now I have the tools I need to handle the bad feelings before they get away from me. I don't have to go down to that bottomless pit again, if I'm careful.

I was just thinking, it has been two years, almost to the day, since my nervous breakdown. Two years…but now, I can finally say with confidence…I am well.

Up the Down Hill

The path goes up.
The path goes down.
The path I walk goes round and round.
The rocks and dips along the way
Belie, confuse, and try to sway,
"This road's too hard,
Too steep, too rough.
Go back! Give up! You're not that tough!"
I'm longing for the moment when
I feel my courage once again.

But deep inside my heart I hear
A Father's plea that help is near.
And so I put my foot again
Upon the road that does not end.

Up the down hill I must climb
While I'm in this land of time.
But in my hand I'm gripping tight
A rod of iron that's glows with light.
It's grit. It's guts.
It's force of will.
That keeps me climbing up that hill.
Up the Down Hill.
Up the Down Hill.

I climb, I sweat,
I feel the pain
That thrusts me down the hill again.
The sky begins to fill with clouds
And covers me with dark, dank shrouds.
The mist I feel is thick and dense.
My mouth feels dry; my brow is tense.
No longer can I see the sky.
I feel it's grown too hard to try.

Then deep inside my heart I hear
A Father's plea that help is near.
And so I put my foot again
Upon the road that does not end.

Up the down hill I must climb
While I'm in this land of time.
But in my hand I'm gripping tight
A rod of iron that's glows with light.
It's grit. It's guts.
It's force of will.
That keeps me climbing up that hill.
Up the Down Hill.
Up the Down Hill.

Epilogue

Life goes on and I'm still on the path to recovery.

Sometimes I get depressed. Other times I'm in a great mood. I'm pretty normal that way and that is good news, indeed.

My saga of self-discovery continues as I have become a student in the most important coursework of my life—how to become a better person. As I have studied, I have learned some techniques that have helped me deal with life in a more effective manner. Some of these techniques include negative thought stopping, meditation, and using art as a means of self-discovery. I still keep journals. I have several, as I discuss different types of issues in each one. Most importantly, I have become "converted" to the value of daily scripture reading and sincere personal prayer. I have to have my time with the Lord. If I don't create this time, I quickly find my life spinning out of control until I manage to pull myself back to what is imperative once again. Christ is the foundation of my very existence.

I am currently working for a major software company. I like my job and the people I work with. I never supposed that I would end up in a job like this, but the Lord's ways truly are magnificent. He knows me better than I know myself.

I guess the most important thing for everyone to know is that I keep going, even when life gets tough. I keep climbing. I get up when I stumble. I just keep moving forward…

Printed in the United States
2226